The
LOW-CARB
Gourmet

Books published by The Random House Publishing Group are available at quantity discounts on bulk purchases for premium, educational, fund-raising, and special sales use. For details, please call 1-800-733-3000.

The
LOW-CARB
Gourmet

A Cookbook for Hungry Dieters

Previously published as *The Low-Carbohydrate Gourmet*

Harriet Brownlee

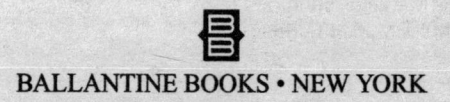

BALLANTINE BOOKS • NEW YORK

Sale of this book without a front cover may be unauthorized. If this book is coverless, it may have been reported to the publisher as "unsold or destroyed" and neither the author nor the publisher may have received payment for it.

A Ballantine Book
Published by The Random House Publishing Group

Copyright © 1974, 2004, copyright renewed 2002 by Harriet Brownlee

All rights reserved under International and Pan-American Copyright Conventions. Published in the United States by Ballantine Books, an imprint of The Random House Publishing Group, a division of Random House, Inc., New York, and simultaneously in Canada by Random House of Canada Limited, Toronto. Originally published in different form as *The Low-Carbohydrate Gourmet* and by William Morrow Company Inc., New York, in 1974.

Grateful acknowledgment is made to the following, for permission to reprint recipe on page 134: Recipe for Steak with Mushroom Sauce from *Annemarie's Personal Cookbook* by Annemarie Huste, copyright © 1968 by Annemarie Huste. Used by permission of The Foley Agency.

Ballantine and colophon are registered trademarks of Random House, Inc.

www.ballantinebooks.com

ISBN 0-345-47176-8

Manufactured in the United States of America

First Mass Market Edition: 1977
Revised Mass Market Edition: 2004

OPM 9 8 7 6 5 4 3 2 1

To all adults who were once fat children, and now, through no fault of their own, must diet for the rest of their lives

Foreword

The excessive eating of carbohydrate foods (sugars and starches) seems to be the current "fat culprit" on the dietary horizon. In my opinion, any dietary regime offering a satisfying approach to the control of carbohydrate intake is not only a welcome addition to the vast number of theories on weight control, but also a sensible approach to good nutrition.

Harriet Brownlee, in *The Low-Carb Gourmet,* offers painlessly sound and sensible methods for low-carbohydrate cooking and eating. She wisely suggests that even with carbohydrate control, food intake should be both reasonably limited and nutritionally safe. Along with her sound advice for subsidizing a low-carbohydrate diet with vitamins and minerals as well as a doctor's supervision, she also provides myriad suggestions for satisfying an addictive "sweet tooth" and for preparing other "unheard-of-on-a-diet" foods with the use of low-carbohydrate substitutes.

Ms. Brownlee discusses the danger of the overenthusiastic claims of most other diets and the possible pitfalls of unsound nutrition even in carefully controlled dietary regimes. She shows how dieters need not resort to fad gimmicks, fad foods, fad recipes—fad diets—in order to lose weight or to maintain one's desired weight.

As a result of her own personal experience in her fight with fatness, she has created a cookbook for dieters that works both to ensure weight loss and to prevent dieting from being a chore or a bore. This book, a needed companion for

Foreword

all those (30 million plus!) in the frequently lonesome world of dieters, is sometimes solemnly, sometimes amusingly, always sensibly written. It is truly a gourmet cookbook—especially for dieters!

—ABRAHAM WEINBERG, M.D.

Acknowledgments

No book is ever solely the work of one person. Many people have influenced me in the writing of this book and I would like to take this opportunity to give them my thanks.

First to my mother, for encouraging and fostering my interest in cooking from childhood and for being my extra pair of hands during the writing of the original version of this book in hardcover; to Dr. Arnold Zentner, for giving me the freedom to create; to Mrs. Shirley Shure, for originally teaching me to bake; to Dr. Robert C. Atkins, for stimulating and fostering my interest in low-carbohydrate cooking; to Dr. Ivor Shapiro, for his gentle encouragement and support throughout the writing of the original book; to Maureen O'Neal, vice president and editorial director at Ballantine Books, for her idea to republish this book; and to Johanna Bowman, who has been such a joy to work with.

Contents

Foreword vii
Acknowledgments ix
Preface xiii
Introduction 3
    Some Sample Menus 11
Tips for Low-Carbohydrate Cooks and Dieters 15
    Tips for Cooks 15
    Some Useful Ingredients for Low-Carbohydrate
        Cooking 17
    Tips for Dieters 24

I   Yes, You Can Bake with Soy Flour   27
II   The Sweet Things in Life   49
III   To Begin a Meal: Hors D'Oeuvres, Appetizers,
        and Soups   99
IV   Meats, The Backbone of Low-
        Carbohydrate Diets   119
V   Fish: Gifts from the Sea   143
VI   Chicken: A Dieter's Best Friend   157
VII   Eggs and Egg Dishes: Thanks to the
        Chickens   173
VIII   Vegetables and Salads: Gifts from the
        Earth   191
IX   A Visit to Asia   219
X   Sauces, Dressings, and Toppings: A Few Little
        Things   249

*Carbohydrate Gram- and Calorie-Counting
  Charts* 265
Index 293

Preface

One of my dreams has always been that medical science would find the way to make me burn all of my food normally and that I would never have to diet again. How many of you have shared that dream with me? To suddenly be able to eat anything you want and not to gain even one pound! Imagine being able to eat without getting fat!

Fat! How I hate that word! I'm sure it is one of the ugliest words in the English language. It even sounds ugly! I think I would rather starve to death than ever allow myself to get fat. Some of you will hate me instantly when you read this, but I am five feet, five inches tall and weight 120 pounds. I can hear you saying already, "How can she write a diet cookbook? How can anyone who's that thin understand what it's like to be fat and have to diet? She's not one of us."

Yes, I am thin. I've been thin all of my adult life. But let me share some of my childhood memories with you. I remember when I was twelve years old and my eighth grade teacher weighed and measured the class and called out the figures for everyone to hear: Harriet Brownlee, five feet tall, 170 pounds. My classmates snickered and laughed at me and how I wished I could hide under my desk or that the floor would open up and I could crawl under it! I pray that teachers don't do that anymore! I remember trying to learn to ride a bicycle and to roller-skate, but being too embarrassed because I was so awkward and so clumsy. I never did learn to do either. I remember when my mother would take me shopping for clothes. "We have nothing here that could possibly fit her. She's too fat. Try another store."

Preface

"No, we have nothing that she could wear here. Why don't you lose weight, dear? You'd be so pretty if you did. Try the chubby department. Maybe they'll have something." I remember how we bought two identical skirts one year, just in different colors. They were the only ones we could get that fit me and my mother was getting disgusted by that time. Were they size 44 or 46? I can't remember, but does it really matter which? I remember graduating from the eighth grade. My mother had to have my graduation dress made for me. It was white organdy. We couldn't find a white dress to fit me in any store. I was the smartest girl in my graduating class. I even had the highest I.Q., but I only remember the sensitive little girl looking out of the window on graduation night with the tears streaming down her face, trying to hide the tears from her family. I was the only pupil in my whole graduating class who didn't get invited to any of the graduation parties, the only one who was completely left out.

I've worn a lot of beautiful designer clothing since those years. I'm a size 8 now. Even though I never learned to roller-skate or to ride a bicycle, in college I learned to swim so gracefully that everyone stops to watch me. And there have been many parties since then, too—parties where I have been the most beautiful young woman in the room. But those childhood memories will be recorded in my mind forever, and even as I wrote about them, the tears were streaming down my face.

This book is my gift to the diet world. The recipes I have included have enabled me to stay on one of the strictest versions of a low-carbohydrate diet for many years—and thus maintain my normal weight. These recipes were originally developed for me because I missed sweets so much. Without them, I doubt that I could have continued such a diet faithfully for such a long time.

I am proud to be able to share my book with you. To give a gift is to give a part of oneself, but for a gift to be valuable, it must be used, not just stored away in a closet. Don't just read the recipes and say, "Umm, that sounds delicious." (And they *are* delicious!) Use these recipes and let them make and keep you thin!

The
LOW-CARB
Gourmet

Introduction

Yes, nobody likes to be fat. But at the same time, nobody, but nobody, likes to diet! We diet simply because we have to. There are those of us whom Fate has willed to be fat, but since fashion and good health dictate that we be thin, we have had to feel exempt from the human race at mealtimes. Worse yet, because diet food has, until now, been so unappetizing, often after we have succeeded in losing a few pounds we have gone back to fattening eating again. Up goes the scale; nobody can spend a lifetime feeling deprived.

Only by acquiring a new eating lifestyle can one *stay* thin. Anyone who has ever had a serious weight problem eventually knows he must diet in some way for the rest of his life, and until medical science discovers a fat-melting pill, dieting will remain the only answer. But how does one go about choosing a diet that allows one to either lose pounds or maintain a low weight, while at the same time allowing him not to feel deprived? Today, the choices of diets are innumerable:

A Complete Starvation Diet: This was the first diet I ever tried and I learned at the young age of thirteen that the only thing this diet would do was make me sick. This isn't just a diet with *bad* nutrition—this one has *no* nutrition!

The Ten-Day Egg Diet or *The Mayo Clinic Diet:* This diet never originated in the Mayo Clinic! After trying it during my college years, I could never again stand the sight of a hardcooked egg. I must admit that it did take some pounds off me in those ten days, but on the tenth day, I promptly passed out. This diet is not only poor nutritionally, it leaves you in a state of constant hunger.

The Old Blitz Diet: By eating cottage cheese and fruit three times a day, you are supposed to take off five pounds in two days. I lost a half pound in four days and was gagging on the cottage cheese by the first night. I didn't mind cottage cheese and fruit for lunch, but for breakfast and dinner, too? Having to eat cottage cheese for dinner, especially on cold winter nights, made me feel inhuman. This diet is psychologically unsatisfying and is also poor nutritionally if you stay on it for any length of time.

The Old Calorie-Counting Diets: I lived with these diets for many years—until I learned better. They did work and even kept me thin. But in order to lose weight or even to maintain my weight, I had to keep my calorie intake so low that not only was I always hungry, I had the worst health of anyone I knew. I had no resistance to disease, took three times as long as anyone else to heal when I got sick, and was always weak and tired. I have iron willpower and rarely break any diet, so I managed to live with low-calorie diets for years. However, I also severely aggravated a case of hypoglycemia—low blood sugar—by always walking around hungry, and came close to losing my life because of it. The damage done during those years can never be completely undone.

If you severely restrict calories all of your life, you cannot get enough basic nutrition to keep you healthy. Besides, most people who aren't as motivated to be thin usually give up when the hunger becomes unbearable.

The Diet Pill Way: Doctors hand these out much too freely! Every doctor I had ever been to, up until the time I met Dr. Robert Atkins, handed me prescriptions for diet pills when I complained I had trouble staying thin. They all assume that you're a glutton and eat too much. Diet pills actually are meant to make you lose weight by suppressing your appetite so that you will cut down your calories. But the minute you stop taking them, your appetite returns in full force. The only way you can stay thin with them is by continuing to take them. Apart from the damage they can do to your body, do you really want to be hooked?

Dr. Stillman's Quick-Weight-Loss Diet: I've known many people who lost weight on this diet, but gained a great amount right back the minute they began to eat normally. Mainly, this diet does not teach good eating habits. Nobody can live on just meat, hard-cooked eggs, cottage cheese, and water for the rest of his or her life. Besides the fact that this is bad nutritionally (I faint on this diet and have known many others who either faint or feel very weak), this diet is boring.

Weight-Watchers Diet: If this diet works for you, use it by all means. It is nutritionally sound and can do you no harm. However, it will not necessarily do you any good either, because it does not work for everyone. I think you may have to be severely overweight to have this diet work for you. I gain weight on it, as do a number of others I've met.

By this time, if you're starting to wonder if the only thing you can do is stay round, take heart. There is still one diet that I have not mentioned. Imagine a diet that lets you eat gourmet meals! Imagine a diet you will be able to stick to when eating in any restaurant! Imagine a diet that does not force you to eat any particular food you do not like! Imagine a diet that lets you have good wines with your dinner! Imagine a diet that lets you lose weight and keep it off forever with just a minimum of willpower! Imagine a diet that's fun!

No, this diet does not exist only in your dreams. It's a diet that you can start living with right now. It's a high-protein, low-carbohydrate diet.

There are many variations of the basic low-carbohydrate diet. The one factor they have in common is that they all restrict carbohydrates but do not restrict calories—hence no hunger. Carbohydrate foods are those that contain high percentages of sugar (which is pure carbohydrate) and starch, including fruits, breads, cakes, candies, pies, soda containing sugar, puddings, cereal, pasta, and some vegetables such as corn and potatoes. Meat, fish, poultry, eggs, butter, oil, margarine, and some mayonnaises contain no carbohydrates while cheeses and salad greens contain only a few.

It's a good idea when starting this diet to equip yourself

with a carbohydrate gram-counting chart. (See the chart on page 268 of this book.) Comprehensive charts are available in any paperback bookshop. *The Doctor's Pocket Calorie, Fat and Carbohydrate Counter* by Allan Borushek is an excellent and very complete paperback book that I found in my local bookstore.

Dr. Atkins' New Carbohydrate Gram Counter is an inexpensive little book that's quite complete, even though it's tiny and easy to slip into a pocket or handbag when going marketing. Another good book to get is the Department of Agriculture Handbook, *Composition of Foods,* which can be obtained by writing to the Government Printing Office in Washington, D.C.

The most liberal of the low-carbohydrate diets was *The Drinking Man's Diet,* otherwise known as *The Air Force Diet.* To follow this diet, you could eat anything you wanted as long as you limited yourself to fewer than 60 grams of carbohydrates per day. There were no limits placed on any other foods. If you lose weight easily, by all means follow this diet. It's the easiest of all.

Dr. Carlton Fredericks was Dr. Robert Atkins's mentor on low-carbohydrate diets. Dr. Fredericks's suggestion that you eat six small meals a day instead of the usual three large ones is excellent and has been recommended to dieters for years. In an article called "Meal Frequency—A Possible Factor in Human Pathology" in *The American Journal of Clinical Nutrition* (August 1970), an experiment is described showing how both men and women, when fed small, frequent meals, were able to eat more than 1,400 calories in excess of the normal intake they needed to maintain their normal weight, without gaining any weight. But when they were fed the same amount of food in two large meals, they gained weight to the degree of their calorie excess.

When it was published, *Dr. Atkins' Diet Revolution* immediately aroused a storm of controversy. One of the biggest criticisms leveled at Dr. Atkins by the American Medical Association was that his diet was too high in saturated fats. I think one of the things that the AMA failed to realize is that by natural selectivity, people will vary their diet. Even if you are allowed to eat eggs, beef, butter, et cetera, you will not necessarily take in too much. Most people want variety in their meals and practically everyone would get sick of eating steaks, roast beef, or very rich food every single day, never mind the cost of these foods in inflationary times.

I do feel that Dr. Atkins should have placed some restrictions on the amounts of food people eat. I'm not saying people should count every calorie, but they should be aware that they shouldn't eat even protein foods out of boredom or unhappiness, for amusement or sociability, or even just because it's mealtime. If you eat only in reasonable quantities, you will not eat an unreasonable amount of fat. And if your doctor advises you, because of your particular state of health, to restrict your intake of saturated fats, many high-protein, low-carbohydrate recipes can be just what you should be using so that you can follow his orders without going on a dreary "I can't eat anything" diet. As a general rule of thumb: The saturated fats people are told to avoid are found in butter, egg yolk, cream cheese and cheeses made from cream or whole milk, sweet or sour cream, beef, lamb, liver, and shrimp. Avoid these and concentrate on egg whites, cheeses made from skim milk or partially skim milk, fish other than shellfish, fowl, veal, and soy flour. Substitute trans-fat-free margarine or olive oil for butter, farmer's cheese for cream cheese, or whipped nonfat dry milk or fat-free half-and-half for heavy cream.

I was Dr. Atkins's patient years ago. I didn't go to him for a diet; I was thin, but I wasn't feeling well. My best friend had just died and I had been going to the hospital every day after work, staying there until eleven P.M. or midnight. She had been like a big sister to me and I wanted to be there for her. I was exhausted after months of this routine. I wasn't really eating properly. Most of the time I was upset when I got home and didn't really feel like eating.

My first visit with Dr. Robert Atkins was an experience. Even though I didn't complain about my weight, he was the only doctor I had ever gone to who was smart enough to take a weight history. He wanted to know what my maximum weight had been and at what age. I told him that I had weighed 170 pounds and was five feet tall at age twelve. He studied me. When he began to speak, I didn't believe what I was hearing. "I admire you more than anyone I've ever met. You're keeping yourself at least a hundred pounds thinner than God intended you to be." Then he raised his voice. "But you're starving to death! You're completely malnourished or you wouldn't look the way you do!" In the weeks that followed, he treated me like a baby that he had to nourish and nurture. He created an individualized diet for me that allowed me to eat a normal amount of food without gaining weight and I did live with the maintenance part of his diet for years. We found that carbohydrates were definitely what threw my weight out of line and that I could not tolerate more than 30 grams of carbohydrate daily without gaining weight. But even with this strict limitation on carbohydrates, I cannot take in unlimited food without having unlimited inches show on my waistline. However, without restricting carbohydrates, I used to have to live on six to seven hundred calories a day—not to lose weight, but just to maintain it.

I will always be grateful to Robert Atkins for diagnosing my hypoglycemia and for taking me off sugar. I'm sure had he not done so, I would be a diabetic today. More doctors should include a five-hour glucose tolerance test as part of their initial workup of a patient and periodically repeat the test. The aim should be to diagnose impaired insulin levels and impaired glucose tolerance before a person becomes a diabetic with the resulting damage that diabetes does to the body. Robert Atkins was truly a pioneer in pointing out the pitfalls of high-carbohydrate diets and for being such a strong advocate of low-carbohydrate diets.

His book *Dr. Atkins' New Diet Revolution* is worth reading, whether you choose to follow his diet or if you prefer one of the other low-carbohydrate diets. It's available in paperback and is an interesting, very well documented book describing some of the latest studies on food, nutrition, low-carbohydrate eating, and exercise. His diet allows the lowest

Introduction

carbs of all of the low-carbohydrate diets but allows a higher saturated-fat content. The jury is still out on the effects of the higher saturated-fat content allowed in his diet, which is why I've chosen to suggest whenever possible eating part–skim milk cheeses for the most part, fat-free half-and-half rather than heavy cream, and using mainly olive oil with just a touch of whipped butter for flavor in my recipes. Only more research in the years to come will give us the answer.

Dr. Arthur Agatston's *The South Beach Diet* is the latest of the low-carbohydrate diets. It is based on the glycemic index, protein, and healthy fats. *The South Beach Diet* is currently on *The New York Times* bestseller list.

The *South Beach Diet: Good Fats, Good Carbs Guide* by Dr. Agatston is a little paperback book that describes his diet, the foods you should eat and those you should stay away from. It's an excellent little book and easy to slip in a pocket or handbag when you go shopping. It gives a lot of information for such a little book. It explains the glycemic index, a trans-fat hot list, which lists foods containing trans fats that you should avoid as they are linked to heart attacks, phases 1 and 2 of his diet, and a list of more than 1,200 foods by category, all in one little book.

All of these books are interesting reading and you'll learn something from all of them. Take that knowledge and choose the diet that you would be comfortable living with, then discuss the diet with your doctor! He should know you and your blood chemistry. Once you've made the choice, then use my recipes to make the diet that you have chosen easier and more pleasant to live with. My recipes are so low in carbohydrates that you should be able to use them with any controlled-carbohydrate diet. Use them and enjoy them!

These recipes are designed to make an easy diet even easier—and much more fun, too. Until now, if you were on a low-carbohydrate diet, you had to accept the fact that even though you never had to bear the torture of walking around hungry all day while dieting, all the foods you enjoyed most were the ones you must give up permanently. You also had to accept the fact that once you reached the weight you desired, these things had to *remain* a part of the past or the pounds would creep right back up on you again. Gone were hot muffins for weekend breakfasts. Gone were cakes and ice cream for snacks and dessert. Gone was the potato salad and the bun for the cheeseburger. Gone, certainly, was anything chocolate. That is, gone until now!

Now, using the recipes I have collected and created, you can eat gourmet meals at home. (How does a dinner of consommé with sherry, glazed rock Cornish hen, tossed salad vinaigrette, and chocolate rum cream roll for dessert sound? The recipes are all in this book.) You can remain on your diet while eating out (with a minimum of study, you'll soon know how to choose carefully), and even enjoy a glass of wine. The chapter that is my greatest pride, "Yes, You Can Bake with Soy Flour," is made up of carefully tested recipes for foods you felt were gone forever: the muffins, pancakes, fancy cakes, and even things chocolate! Imagine good-tasting food that's good for you—both nutritionally and dietetically.

Just so you will get a look at how scrumptious it is all going to be, and so you can begin planning low-carbohydrate menus of your own, I have compiled the following sample menus for breakfast, brunch, lunch, and dinner. Enjoy your new, thin lifestyle; enjoy the new, thin you!

Some Sample Menus

Breakfast

1. Cheese and Herb Omelet
   Hot Coffee or Tea
2. Cheddar Scrambled Eggs
   Sausage
   Hot Coffee or Tea
3. Broiled Canadian Bacon
   Easy-Mix Muffins with Whipped Butter and Sugarless Strawberry Jam
   Hot Coffee or Tea
4. Double-Cheese Omelet
   Cinnamon-Pecan Puffins
   Hot Coffee or Tea

Brunch

1. Fresh Strawberries with Fat-Free Half-and-Half
   A Favorite Omelet
   Easy-Mix Muffins
   Hot Coffee or Tea
2. Cantaloupe Wedges with Fresh Mint
   Ham-Mushroom Omelet
   Cinnamon-Pecan Puffins
   Hot Coffee or Tea
3. Mushroom Soufflé Omelet
   Broiled Canadian Bacon
   Cinnamon Bread with Light Variety Cream Cheese and Sugarless Jam
   Hot Coffee or Tea
4. Easy-Mix Pancakes with Whipped Butter and Sugarless Maple Syrup or Jam
   Sausage
   Hot Coffee or Tea

5. French Toast with Sugarless Maple Syrup or Jam
   Broiled Canadian Bacon
   Hot Coffee or Tea
   Ham Omelet
   Cinnamon Bread with Nutted Light Variety Cream
     Cheese
   Hot Coffee or Tea

Lunch

1. Salade Niçoise
   Lemon Cake-Pudding
   Iced Coffee or Tea
2. Mushroom, Herb, and Cheese Omelet
   Tossed Lettuce and Tomato Salad with Oil, Vinegar,
     and Garlic Dressing
   Raspberry Sponge Pudding
3. Cheese-Filled Hamburgers
   Potato-like Salad
   Sugarless Soda
4. Curried Chicken Salad on a Bed of Lettuce
   Cantaloupe Wedges
   Iced or Hot Tea
5. French Omelet Filled with Chicken Liver Sauté
   Tossed Green Salad with Vinaigrette Dressing
   Easy-Mix Muffins with Whipped Butter (served hot)
   Chocolate Almond Pudding

Dinner

1. Cold Shrimp with Dilled Shrimp Sauce
   Consommé with Sherry
   Glazed Rock Cornish Hens
   Tossed Salad with Garlic-Flavored Vinaigrette
     Dressing
   Chocolate Rum Cream Roll
   Hot Coffee or Tea
2. Cold Strawberry Soup

Introduction 13

    Steak with Mushroom and Wine Sauce
    Green Beans Amandine
    Bibb Lettuce and Tomato Salad with Roquefort or
       Vinaigrette Dressing
    Lemon Cream Roll
    Coffee or Spiced Tea

3. Fresh Mushroom Soup (hot in winter or cold in summer)
   Broiled Chicken with Shallot Butter
   Tossed Green Salad with Roquefort Dressing
   Strawberry or Chocolate Ice Cream
   Hot or Iced Coffee or Tea

4. Hot Onion Soup
   Chicken Beauvais
   Green Beans Amandine
   Tossed Salad with Garlic-Flavored Vinaigrette Dressing
   Lemon Chiffon Pie with Brazil Nut Crust
   Hot Coffee or Tea

5. Greek Lemon Soup
   Lamb Shish Kebab
   Strawberry Ice Cream
   Hot Coffee

6. Melon with Prosciutto
   Beef Stroganoff
   Tossed Salad with Garlic-Flavored Vinaigrette Dressing
   Strawberry Granite
   Hot Coffee or Tea

7. Assorted Cold Hors d'Oeuvres
   Party Veal Scallops
   Braised Endive
   Lemon Mousse with Strawberries
   Hot Coffee or Tea

8. Cold Lemon Sorrel Soup
   Shad en Papillote
   Braised Celery
   Tomato Salad

14 THE LOW-CARB GOURMET

    Chocolate Mousse
    Iced or Hot Coffee

9. Meat-Crusted Pizza
   Tossed Green Salad with Vinaigrette Dressing
   Vanilla or Chocolate Ice Cream
   Hot Coffee or Tea

10. Apricot-Glazed Turkey London Broil
    Cauliflower with Cheese
    Tossed Green Salad with Garlic-Flavored Vinaigrette
      Dressing
    Jelly Roll with Apricot Jam Filling
    Hot Coffee or Tea

Tips for Low-Carbohydrate Cooks and Dieters

Tips for Cooks

1. Experiment with different blends of coffee. Jamaican Blue Mountain coffee is superb although expensive, as is Hawaiian Kona coffee. Chocolate hazelnut and chocolate almond coffees are delicious, especially if you're a chocoholic. They're available as decaf also.
2. Experiment with different types of tea. There are black teas scented with fruit flavors such as strawberry, raspberry, mango, et cetera. Most of the time I don't even need to sweeten these.
3. Concentrate on the following low-carbohydrate vegetables when planning your menus: asparagus, mushrooms, spinach, cucumbers, green beans, celery, cauliflower, zucchini, endives, escarole, and peppers. These vegetables are also low in calories and contain needed vitamins and minerals. Beware of high-carbohydrate vegetables such as corn, peas, lima beans, beets, and both white and sweet potatoes.
4. The best buys in low-carbohydrate fruit are berries of all kinds, apricots, peaches, rhubarb, and tangerines. These fruits are also low on the glycemic index. Melons of all kinds are low-carbohydrate but are a little higher on the glycemic index (although not watermelon).
5. If buying filleted fish and you cannot judge its freshness, press the fleshiest part of the fish with your finger. If it leaves a dent that does not spring back quickly, the fish is not fresh. Do not buy it.

6. Herbs de Provence is a dried-herb mixture from France that is used to flavor meats, sauces, salads, and even pizza. It's a mixture of thyme, basil, savory, fennel, and lavender flowers. If not available in a gourmet food store near you, the mixture can be ordered from Zabar's, one of my favorite shops in New York. Order online at www.zabars.com or call 212-787-2000.
7. Poissonnade is a dried-herb mixture from France that is used primarily to flavor fish. It consists of fennel seeds, marjoram, savory, sage, and thyme. I actually like to use this mixture for lamb also. Like herbs de Provence, this too can be ordered from Zabar's, if not available near you.
8. If you do not have a greengrocer near you or a good fruit and vegetable store that sells fresh herbs, start a little herb garden on a sunny window. If you haven't got a sunny window, herbs can easily be grown under lights. I once had herbs growing on a bookshelf under lights. They're very easy to grow; just keep them well watered. A basic herb garden might consist of basil, tarragon, thyme, rosemary, chive, chervil, and mint. It's great to just pick the herbs you want to use from your little garden.
9. Beware of most bottled salad dressings, including imitation mayonnaise, even the low-calorie and dietetic ones. They are fairly high in carbohydrates. Concentrate on the salad dressing recipes in this book, and, with regard to mayonnaise, I'd suggest Hellmann's. Balsamic vinegar and olive oil with a little fresh garlic is wonderful as a salad dressing. Olive oil and fresh lemon juice also make a good dressing. Use 2 to 3 parts oil to 1 part vinegar or lemon juice.
10. To save money, buy a roast of beef and have the butcher cut it into steaks. A whole fillet of beef is a good buy when it is on sale.
11. Liver and other organ meats may be high in iron, but they are also high in carbohydrates. Beware, also, of processed meats that are made with corn syrup.

Tips for Low-Carbohydrate Cooks and Dieters 17

12. Measure or weigh soy flour in a plastic bag. Add the baking powder and salt to the bag and then sift all dry ingredients directly into the liquid. A paper plate is handy to weigh dry and wet ingredients.
13. A kitchen scale is invaluable. Most kitchen scales give weight in both ounces and grams so you can have a precise idea of exactly how many grams of carbohydrates you will be consuming. Measuring by weight is the most accurate way to measure and is much easier than measuring with cups.
14. Get out of the kitchen if you are overtired and rest for a little while. Otherwise, the only thing you will succeed in doing is having an accident or ruining something you are attempting to prepare. You may even find yourself nibbling unnecessarily!

Some Useful Ingredients for Low-Carbohydrate Cooking

Artificial Sweeteners

Artificial sweeteners are available in granulated, liquid, and tablet forms. For many of the recipes in this book, granulated sweetener is a must. It is available from various companies, but be careful, as some brands contain more carbohydrates than others. This must be taken into account when counting the carbohydrate gram content of a recipe. My favorite sweetener for my recipes is sucralose, which is marketed under the name Splenda®. For my tea or coffee, I like to use an envelope of Splenda® and an envelope of Sweet'n Low together. It just seems to taste better to me when I mix the two. They are both considered safe by the FDA.

A brown sugar substitute is also available under the name Brown Sugar Twin and it is quite good. I've used it in a few recipes in this book.

Cheeses

Swiss Gruyère Cheese. I have used imported Swiss Gruyère cheese in a number of recipes in this book. This is not the processed Gruyère like Swiss Knight or other wedged types, but is a cheese similar to Swiss Emmenthal with small holes and a nutty flavor. It's marvelous for cooking as well as for eating.

Parmesan Cheese. Buy imported Italian Parmesan cheese in a chunk and grate it freshly in your blender or food processor whenever you need it. Parmesan cheese may be stored in the freezer.

Ricotta Cheese. This is the Italian form of cottage cheese. It is unsalted and is used for Italian cheesecakes and Italian pastries such as cannoli. Because it is smooth and delicious, I have used it as a filling for my cream roll cakes and to take the place of ice cream in milk shakes. It absorbs flavorings very well. The part-skim variety is just as good as the full-fat variety.

Farmer's Cheese. This is a pressed cottage cheese. The advantage of using farmer's cheese rather than cottage cheese is that because the water has been pressed out, such dishes as cheesecake and blintzes are not too moist.

Chinese and Japanese Ingredients (Specialties)

Tofu. These little cakes of bean curd are made from soybeans and are an inexpensive source of protein. They absorb flavor well and are particularly suited to the taste of soy sauce. Use them in making sukiyaki or cut them into cubes, dip them in soy sauce, and use as a Chinese hors d'oeuvre.

Chinese Celery or Bok Choy. This vegetable is a cross between celery and cabbage. It is becoming increasingly popular and can now be found in fruit and vegetable stores and supermarkets as well as in Chinatown. Use it as a vegetable in Chinese stir-fried dishes or in a salad.

Chinese Dried Mushrooms. These marvelous thick, meaty mushrooms are only available in Chinese specialty shops,

Tips for Low-Carbohydrate Cooks and Dieters

but are definitely worth seeking out. As a substitute, you can use Japanese dried mushrooms, but they are not as meaty. They will keep well without refrigeration in an airtight container. Use them in Chinese stir-fried dishes.

Chinese Five-Spice Powder. This spice is available only in Chinese specialty shops. If you do not have access to one, combine equal parts of powdered cinnamon, powdered cloves, powdered aniseed, and thyme. (Only four spices, but the taste is similar.) It is a delicious addition to Chinese roast pork.

Chinese Sesame Oil. This is available in any Asian food shop, Japanese or Chinese, and is *not* the same as the sesame oil found in health food stores. Use it in Chinese-style salad dressings.

Rice Vinegar. Rice vinegar is used for Chinese and Japanese recipes. Kikkoman rice vinegar is excellent and is available in supermarkets. A trip to any Asian food store will yield other appropriate brands.

Sake. This is a Japanese rice wine and is used in Japanese recipes. It is available in any liquor store. A dry sherry can be used as a substitute.

Soy Sauce. Buy imported soy sauce because the American soy sauce is far too salty. Chinese soy sauce is now coming into the United States from mainland China and is absolutely delicious. Japanese Kikkoman soy sauce is also very good and is available in all supermarkets. Use it if the Chinese soy sauce is unavailable. See my recipe for Chinese Salad Dressing, page 223, for an interesting use for soy sauce. Use the lower-salt varieties whenever possible. We are all under too much stress now, and we do not want our blood pressure to get too high.

Chives

Fresh chives are a delicious addition to eggs, cottage cheese, meats, and poultry, among other things. Chives are available frozen or dried, but fresh are the best and can be bought at good fruit and vegetable markets. Chop them, place them in an airtight plastic container, and freeze them yourself. If you have a sunny window, try growing them in little pots. They require very little attention since they are basically a weed.

Cornstarch

I've used very tiny amounts of cornstarch in my Chinese recipes, but one teaspoon of cornstarch contains 2.3 grams of carbohydrate. If you do not want to use these few extra grams, you may always eliminate the cornstarch.

Cream of Tartar

Unless you own a copper bowl for beating egg whites, always add ¼ teaspoon of cream of tartar for every two egg whites you beat. The cream of tartar adds the needed acidity that helps stabilize the egg whites so that they beat more easily and retain their firmness.

Curry Powder

Even if you've never liked curry before, try experimenting with various brands because each one has a different taste and you may find one that you like. My favorite is an imported Madras curry powder produced under the Sun Brand label.

Dill

Fresh dill is available in all good fruit and vegetable markets. Dried dill weed can be obtained in jars, but fresh dill is far more delicious.

Eggs

Eggs are one of the best buys in protein. Buy the freshest eggs possible. Test an egg's freshness by immersing it in cold water. If it lies flat, it is very fresh; if it sits up, it is not fresh and should not be eaten. Anything in between may be used for baking, but I don't suggest using it for an egg dish. Store

Tips for Low-Carbohydrate Cooks and Dieters

eggs in the refrigerator, then to bring to room temperature, immerse them in warm water for 5 to 10 minutes.

Extracts

Extracts are available in a wide variety of flavors. Different brands differ in taste, so experiment. Wagner's has an excellent selection including such flavors as chocolate, banana, raspberry, mocha, coconut, et cetera. Ehler's has good extracts as does McCormick, and these are available in local markets. Wagner's is available in specialty food stores. You can order online from one of the best New York food stores at www.zabars.com or call them at 212-787-2000.

Food Coloring

Food coloring is available in all supermarkets. It is completely harmless and completely tasteless. Just follow the directions on the box for the color you desire.

Gingerroot and Ginger Juice

Fresh gingerroot is available in all supermarkets. In the fall, the young ginger comes into season and it, with its delicate flavor, is my favorite. Fresh ginger can be stored in dry sherry in an airtight container placed in the refrigerator. It will keep indefinitely. I have had success freezing it also, but I prefer it stored in sherry. Ginger juice is made by squeezing the fresh gingerroot through a garlic press. The resulting ginger juice is excellent when used in Chinese stir-fried dishes or Chinese salad dressing.

Mayonnaise

Mayonnaise and salad dressing are not the same. Either you can make your own mayonnaise or buy Hellmann's on the east coast or Best Foods on the west coast. These contain the least sugar.

Mushrooms

Buy only firm, crisp, closed white mushrooms. When mushrooms are brown or open it means they have been sitting around too long. Mushrooms should not be washed. If they are closed, it will not be necessary. They should be wiped with a damp paper towel or damp cloth only. If you've never eaten raw mushrooms, by all means try them! Porcini and portobello mushrooms are wonderful and meaty.

Oil

For salads, I like good-quality olive oil. Bertolli and Colavita are both excellent brands. Health food stores carry a cold pressed garlic and oil that tastes good, too. Peanut oil is used for Chinese cooking and is available in any supermarket.

Pam and Other Cooking Sprays

Pam and other cooking sprays such as an olive oil spray are the latest marvels to come to the market shelves. Spray any pan with one of these sprays and it will keep food from sticking, consequently allowing you to use less butter or oil in a recipe. It's particularly good for muffin pans, cake pans, et cetera.

Prosciutto

This is Italian smoked ham. It is customarily sliced into very thin slices and used in many Italian recipes or as an appetizer wrapped around cantaloupe wedges. If it is unavailable, a mild Westphalian ham may be substituted.

Shallots

Shallots are a cross between garlic and onions. They are used a great deal in French cooking. If they are unavailable, onions may be substituted.

Tips for Low-Carbohydrate Cooks and Dieters 23

Sherry

Use either an Amontillado sherry or a Fino sherry when a recipe calls for dry sherry. I use a high-quality sherry; only a small amount is needed, so it is not very expensive to use the best.

Soy Flour

Soy flour is available in all health food stores and many supermarkets. My recipes call for full-fat soy flour, which has the least amount of carbohydrates. It is also available toasted, but I don't particularly like it. The advantage of soy flour over wheat flour is that soy flour has a high protein content and a very low carbohydrate content. Arrowhead Mills and Red Mill were the two brands I found best. See my Seasoned Soy Flour recipe, page 29.

Stock—Chicken or Beef

Canned chicken stock and beef stock are the best substitutes for homemade. Bouillon cubes or powder may also be used, but they are usually too salty. Always buy the low-sodium variety.

Sugarless Diet Jams

Be careful when buying sugarless jams. Some brands are made with sorbitol, which is not a carbohydrate-free sweetener. It just metabolizes more slowly than sugar. I suggest either Smucker's, Polaner's, or Steel's sugarless preserves. Steel's is the lowest in carbs of the three, but not as easily available. They come in a wide variety of flavors and are very good. I've used them a number of times in my recipes.

Vinegar

Always buy good-quality vinegar. For salads, imported wine vinegar is the best because it's the mildest and most delicate-tasting. It is available in some supermarkets as well as in gourmet specialty shops and can be purchased flavored with shallots, garlic, tarragon, lemon, and even champagne. Rice vinegar is used for Chinese and Japanese recipes. See Chinese and Japanese Ingredients (Specialties), page 18. Balsamic vinegar can make almost anything taste good, be it a salad or as part of a sauce.

Wine

Either American or French wines may be used. I generally prefer to use French dry vermouth in place of white wine as wine keeps only for two or three days, even in the refrigerator, and then turns to vinegar. Dry vermouth keeps indefinitely in the refrigerator.

Tips for Dieters

1. If you are dying for something sweet and on the verge of breaking your diet, take a tablespoonful or two of artificially sweetened jam or put a little artificial sweetener on your tongue. It will kill the craving.
2. Read labels carefully. There are hidden carbohydrates in many foods.
3. Beware of hidden carbohydrates when eating in restaurants. A friend of mine ruined her diet for months by eating generous amounts of the bottled orange-colored French dressing served in many restaurants because she thought it had no carbohydrates, not realizing it is only the oil-and-vinegar French dressing that has no carbohydrates.
4. Always leave yourself a little hungry when you leave the table and wait for at least an hour before you eat anything else. By that time, your blood sugar may have risen enough so that you'll no longer need any more food.
5. Always eat something before you go to someone's house for dinner if you don't know what is being served. This

Tips for Low-Carbohydrate Cooks and Dieters

will keep you from eating fattening food just because you're hungry or because there's nothing else to eat.
6. Always choose the lowest carbohydrate foods and beverages. You get more mileage that way.
7. If you're angry or upset, take a long walk or go to sleep instead of heading for the refrigerator. I'm lucky in this respect—when I'm upset I can't eat or stand the smell of food.
8. Become a gourmet. Eat only food that tastes really superb.
9. If you find you simply must nibble on something, try to keep cold meat and chicken, cooked lobster, shrimp, and crabmeat, low-fat cheese, or a hard-cooked egg on hand for just such emergencies. When preparing dinner, cook a little extra to save for snacks.
10. Always check with your doctor before embarking on any diet or dietary regime. Make sure to take the correct vitamin and mineral supplements that he or she prescribes in order to meet minimum daily requirements.

I.

Yes, You Can Bake with Soy Flour

Seasoned Soy Flour 29
Batter for Frying 30
Easy-Mix Muffins 31
Easy-Mix Muffins—A Variation 32
Cinnamon-Pecan Puffins 32
Cinnamon Bread 33
Cinnamon-Nut Coffee Cake Squares 34
Pecan Butter Coffee Cake 35
Easy-Mix Pancakes 36
Puffy Pancakes 37
French Toast 38
Basic Noodle Dough 39
Herbed Rolls 40
Parmesan Puffs 41
Sweet Crêpes 42
Sponge Cake Cream Rolls 43
Gingerbread Squares 45
Brazil Nut Pie Crust 46
Sweet Pie Crust 47

Yes, You Can Bake with Soy Flour

This chapter is my pride and joy!

Everybody has always said that it was impossible to bake using soy flour alone. These recipes prove everybody was wrong. It can be done. The advantage of using soy flour is that it is very high in protein and very low in carbohydrates. However, if it were used interchangeably with regular flour, the finished product would be so heavy that it would leave a lump in your stomach. One of the problems in developing these recipes was to make baked goods as light as those made with regular flour. I think you will agree that I succeeded.

Seasoned Soy Flour

Use this seasoned soy flour whenever a recipe calls for seasoned flour.

Makes ¼ cup

30 grams (¼ cup, unsifted) full-fat soy flour
½ teaspoon salt
2 dashes garlic powder
2 dashes onion powder
2 dashes ground celery seed
¼ teaspoon freshly ground black pepper

Combine all ingredients, mix thoroughly, and place in an airtight container. Set aside to use as needed.

9.1 grams of carbohydrate in entire recipe; makes ¼ cup, each tablespoon containing 2.9 grams of carbohydrate.

Batter for Frying

Makes ½ cup

2 extra-large eggs, at room temperature, separated
¼ teaspoon cream of tartar
15 grams (2 tablespoons) full-fat soy flour
⅛ teaspoon baking powder
⅛ teaspoon salt
⅛ teaspoon ground celery seed
⅛ teaspoon black pepper
Few dashes of onion powder
2 tablespoons grated Parmesan cheese

Beat egg whites until foamy, add cream of tartar, and continue beating until whites are stiff but not dry. Beat egg yolks, then gently fold into whites. Combine soy flour with baking powder, salt, and spices and sift into eggs. Fold in gently. Fold in the Parmesan cheese.

6.0 grams of carbohydrate in entire recipe.

NOTE: Use this as a batter for either deep or shallow frying. Try deep-frying vegetables such as zucchini, eggplant, or any other ingredients commonly used in a *Fritto misto*. If desired, ingredients can be coated with additional grated Parmesan cheese before coating with batter.

Easy-Mix Muffins

These are so easy to make that even my friends who can't cook can make them.

Makes 12 muffins

90 grams (about ¾ cup, unsifted) full-fat soy flour
1 tablespoon baking powder
Dash of salt
3 extra-large eggs
¼ cup fat-free half-and-half
½ cup plus 1 tablespoon cold water
¼ teaspoon nutmeg, freshly grated
1½ teaspoons butter extract
1½ teaspoons vanilla extract
Granulated artificial sweetener equal to 6 tablespoons sugar

Preheat oven to 400° F. Combine soy flour, baking powder, and salt and set aside. (I usually weigh the flour in a plastic bag, add the other ingredients and then set the bag aside.) Beat eggs thoroughly, then add the half-and-half, water, nutmeg, extracts, and sweetener. Sift in the soy flour mixture and beat until well combined. The texture should resemble sour cream.

Either grease muffin tins or fill muffin tins with special papers designed for them and divide mixture into 12 muffins. Top with Cinnamon-Sugar Topping (page 262) if desired. Bake the muffins for 17 to 20 minutes or till done. Store in the refrigerator in a plastic bag when cooled. These muffins freeze beautifully and can easily be reheated in aluminum foil.

36.0 grams of carbohydrate in entire recipe; makes 12 muffins, each muffin containing 3.0 grams of carbohydrate.

Easy-Mix Muffins—A Variation

Follow the recipe for Easy-Mix Muffins, adding in ¼ teaspoon of cinnamon and ¼ teaspoon of almond extract with the other flavorings.

Cinnamon-Pecan Puffins

Puffins are a cross between a popover and a muffin. If you've been dreaming of hot popovers, here's a worthy substitute!

Makes 8 puffins

1½ ounces pecans
½ teaspoon cinnamon
Granulated artificial sweetener equal to 1 tablespoon sugar
3 extra-large eggs, at room temperature, separated
¼ teaspoon cream of tartar
3 tablespoons sour cream, 50 percent reduced fat
¾ teaspoon butter extract
½ teaspoon vanilla extract
20 drops bitter almond extract
3 tablespoons cold water
Granulated artificial sweetener equal to ⅛ cup sugar
30 grams (¼ cup, unsifted) full-fat soy flour
¾ teaspoon baking powder
Dash of salt

Chop nuts (easily done in a blender or a food processor). Combine with cinnamon and granulated artificial sweetener equal to 1 tablespoon sugar and mix thoroughly. Set aside for topping.

Preheat oven to 325° F. Separate eggs. Beat egg whites with cream of tartar until stiff but not dry. Beat egg yolks till thick and lemon-colored. To egg yolks, add sour cream, extracts, artificial sweetener equal to ⅛ cup sugar, and water and beat thoroughly. Combine soy flour, baking powder, and salt and sift into the yolk mixture. Stir until combined, then gently fold in the egg whites.

Grease a muffin or cupcake tin for 8 puffins. Spoon 1 tablespoon of batter into each greased section. Sprinkle a little topping mixture over this batter, then spoon in remaining batter, dividing it evenly. Top with remaining nut mixture and bake in preheated oven for 50 to 60 minutes. Cool the puffins completely in the pan (even if it takes a few hours). To store, place in refrigerator in a plastic bag with 3 tiny holes punctured on each side. (Use a paring knife or fork to make the holes.) To reheat, place in moderate oven for 8 to 10 minutes.

21.6 grams of carbohydrate in entire recipe; when making 8 puffins, each puffin contains 2.7 grams of carbohydrate.

NOTE: For puffins with the texture of popovers, use 3 tablespoons water; for a muffin texture, use 2 tablespoons water.

Cinnamon Bread

Makes 4 small loaves

Nonfat, nonstick cooking spray (page 22)
Butter or shortening for greasing
30 grams (¼ cup, unsifted) full-fat soy flour
½ teaspoon baking powder
Dash of salt
6 extra-large eggs, at room temperature, separated
¼ teaspoon cream of tartar
2 tablespoons cold water
1 teaspoon cinnamon
Granulated artificial sweetener equal to 6 tablespoons sugar
2 teaspoons butter extract

Preheat oven to 350° F. Prepare 4 small bread pans, each measuring 6 × 3½ × 2 inches, by coating with cooking spray and greasing lightly. Set aside.

Sift together soy flour, baking powder, and salt and set aside. Beat egg whites until foamy, add cream of tartar, and continue beating until stiff but not dry. Beat yolks until thick and lemon-colored. To the yolks add water, cinnamon, artificial sweetener, and butter extract, beating until thoroughly combined. Sift in soy flour mixture and beat again until smooth. Fold a little of the beaten egg whites into the yolk mixture and blend thoroughly. Then very gently fold in remaining whites, being careful not to break them down.

Divide batter among the prepared pans. Place the pans in the oven and bake 1 hour. Store loaves in the refrigerator in a plastic bag, punctured with 2 or 3 small holes on each side. To serve, slice each loaf in 8 slices. Try this bread with Nutted Cheese Spread (page 263) or with fat-reduced cream cheese and sugarless strawberry jam.

12.8 grams of carbohydrate in entire recipe; makes 4 loaves of bread, each loaf containing 3.2 grams of carbohydrate. Assuming 8 slices of bread per loaf, each slice contains 0.4 grams of carbohydrate.

NOTE: This recipe can easily be cut in half, but as long as you are making it, it is easier to make more and freeze loaves that will not be used immediately.

Cinnamon-Nut Coffee Cake Squares

Makes 12 squares

15 grams (⅛ cup, unsifted) soy flour
¾ teaspoon baking powder
1¼ teaspoons ground cinnamon
Dash of salt
3 extra-large eggs, at room temperature, separated

Yes, You Can Bake with Soy Flour 35

¼ teaspoon cream of tartar
4 tablespoons sour cream, 50 percent reduced fat
Granulated artificial sweetener equal to ½ cup plus
  1 tablespoon sugar
½ teaspoon vanilla extract
½ teaspoon butter extract
½ cup finely chopped pecans or walnuts
1 tablespoon melted butter and 1 tablespoon extra-virgin
  olive oil

Preheat oven to 350° F. Combine soy flour, baking powder, cinnamon, and salt and set aside. Beat egg whites until frothy, add cream of tartar, and continue beating till stiff but not dry. In another bowl, beat egg yolks at high speed with an electric mixer until thick and lemon-colored (about 5 minutes). Add to the yolks the sour cream, sweetener, and extracts and beat 1 to 2 minutes more. Sift in soy flour mixture and beat till smooth. Gently fold in the egg whites and then the nuts. Pour batter into a greased 8-inch square pan and bake for 5 minutes. Drizzle melted butter and oil mixture over the cake and bake for another 50 to 55 minutes. Cool cake, then cut into squares.

22.8 grams of carbohydrate in entire recipe if made with walnuts. Makes 12 squares, each square containing 1.9 grams of carbohydrate.
20.4 grams of carbohydrate in entire recipe if made with pecans, and 1.7 grams of carbohydrate per square.

Pecan Butter Coffee Cake

Makes 18 squares

1 recipe Butter Sponge Cake (page 43)
⅔ cup finely chopped pecans
Granulated artificial sweetener equal to ¼ cup sugar
½ teaspoon ground cinnamon

Preheat oven to 325° F. Thoroughly grease a 13 × 9 × 2-inch cake pan. Pour in approximately half of the prepared cake batter. Combine chopped pecans, artificial sweetener, and cinnamon and sprinkle half of the pecan mixture evenly over the batter. Pour in remaining batter and sprinkle with remaining nut mixture. Bake 35 to 40 minutes or until cake tests done. Cool cake in the pan, then cut into squares. Place squares in a plastic bag punctured with 2 or 3 holes and refrigerate overnight to improve texture.

21.6 grams of carbohydrate in entire recipe; if making 18 squares, each square contains 1.2 grams of carbohydrate.

NOTE: Half of this recipe is perfect for an 8-inch square pan and makes 9 squares.

Easy-Mix Pancakes

Makes approximately 20 pancakes

90 grams (¾ cup, unsifted) full-fat soy flour
1 tablespoon baking powder
3 extra-large eggs
¼ cup fat-free half-and-half
¾ cup plus 2 tablespoons cold water
1½ teaspoons butter extract
1½ teaspoons vanilla extract
Generous dash of nutmeg
Artificial sweetener equal to 2 tablespoons sugar
Butter and light olive oil for frying

Combine soy flour and baking powder and set aside. Beat eggs thoroughly, then add half-and-half, water, extracts, nutmeg, and sweetener. Sift in the soy flour mixture and beat until well combined. Grease a griddle with a tablespoon of butter and oil and heat until a few drops of water sizzle when splashed on it. Drop the batter onto the griddle with a soup ladle. When the pancakes are puffed and full of bubbles, turn them, and brown the other side. Finished pancakes may be kept warm in a 200° F. oven. Serve hot with butter and sugarless syrup or sugarless jam.

36.0 grams of carbohydrate in entire recipe; makes approximately 20 pancakes, each pancake containing 1.8 grams of carbohydrate.

NOTE: These pancakes can be made in larger quantities in advance and frozen, wrapped in aluminum foil. Simply rewarm them in a moderate oven.

Puffy Pancakes

Makes 20 pancakes

30 grams (¼ cup, unsifted) full-fat soy flour
¾ teaspoon baking powder
Dash of salt
4 extra-large eggs, at room temperature, separated
½ teaspoon cream of tartar
1 cup pot cheese
½ teaspoon vanilla extract
1 teaspoon butter extract
2 dashes cinnamon
2 dashes nutmeg
2 teaspoons water
Granulated artificial sweetener equal to 2 tablespoons sugar
Butter and light olive oil for frying

Mix the flour, baking powder, and salt together and set aside. Separate eggs, placing yolks in a blender or food processor and whites in a bowl. Add cream of tartar to the egg whites and beat until stiff but not dry. To the yolks, add the pot cheese and remaining ingredients and blend until smooth. Empty the cheese-yolk mixture into beaten egg whites and sift the flour mixture over that. Gently fold everything together.

Heat a griddle and grease it lightly. Drop batter from the tip of a large spoon onto the griddle. Bake over a low flame until pancake rises and surface is dotted with bubbles. Turn and bake the second side until golden brown. While making second and third batches, keep the finished pancakes hot in a warm oven (about 200° F.). Serve hot with sugar-free syrup or sugar-free jam.

17.9 grams of carbohydrate in entire recipe; if making 20 pancakes, each pancake contains 0.9 grams of carbohydrate.

NOTE: These pancakes can be wrapped in aluminum foil and frozen, then rewarmed in a moderate oven. They lose a little of their original puffiness, but are still good, especially for days when you are in a hurry.

French Toast

Makes 2 servings of 4 pieces each

1 loaf Cinnamon Bread (page 33)
1 egg
3 tablespoons fat-free half-and-half
3 tablespoons cold water
¼ teaspoon vanilla extract
Generous dash of freshly ground nutmeg
2 tablespoons very light olive oil and 2 teaspoons whipped butter for frying

Slice the bread into 8 slices. Beat egg thoroughly, then beat in the half-and-half, water, vanilla, and nutmeg. Dip bread slices in the egg mixture one at a time. Spread half of the butter and oil on a nonstick grill and fry the bread until golden brown on first side. Turn the slices, add a little extra butter and oil under each, and brown the second side. Serve hot with sugarless maple syrup or sugarless diet jam.

8.4 grams of carbohydrate in entire recipe; if serving 2, each 4-slice serving contains 4.2 grams of carbohydrate.

Basic Noodle Dough

Miss your fettuccine? It's not forbidden anymore.

Makes 4 servings

2 extra-large eggs, at room temperature, separated
60 grams (½ cup, unsifted) full-fat soy flour
2 teaspoons salt
15 grams (2 tablespoons, unsifted) additional soy flour
3 quarts water

Beat eggs thoroughly with a fork or wire whisk. Add soy flour and half a teaspoon of salt and mix well. Place a large sheet of waxed paper on a flat surface, or use a wooden board, if you have one. Sift a tiny amount of the extra soy flour all over the waxed paper or board. Place the dough on the waxed paper, making sure that all surfaces, top and bottom, get a light coating of the soy flour. Roll out the dough with a rolling pin until very thin. (I like the French rolling pins without any handles best.) Try to roll the dough into a rectangular shape. Work fast!

Beginning with the narrow end, gently fold over about 2 inches of dough and continue turning like a jelly roll until the roll is about 3 inches thick. Dough should be dry enough so layers do not stick together, but should not have a heavy coating of extra soy flour. With a very sharp knife, cut rolled dough in even slices—¼-inch wide for fettuccine and as desired for other pasta. Unroll strips carefully so as not to break them, and arrange on waxed paper, keeping flat. The noodles may be left to dry for 1 or 2 hours, or cooked immediately.

To cook, bring water to a rolling boil. Add remainder of salt and put in the pasta, pushing it down gently until all is submerged in the water. (A little oil added will keep the pasta from sticking.) Cook to the al dente stage, testing frequently to make sure the pasta does not overcook. (*Al dente* means tender but still firm to bite.) Drain pasta thoroughly in a colander and use it with your favorite pasta recipe.

23.8 grams of carbohydrate in entire recipe; if serving 4, each serving contains 6.0 grams of carbohydrate.

Herbed Rolls

Try these rolls filled with chicken salad.

Makes 6 rolls

3 extra-large eggs, at room temperature, separated
¼ teaspoon cream of tartar
4 tablespoons cottage cheese
¼ teaspoon ground celery seed
¼ teaspoon salt
2 dashes white pepper
¼ teaspoon dill weed
Nonfat, nonstick cooking spray
½ teaspoon poppy seeds

Preheat oven to 300° F. Beat egg whites until foamy, add cream of tartar, and continue beating until stiff but not dry. Mix together egg yolks, cottage cheese, celery seed, salt, pepper, and dill weed. Very gently fold the yolk mixture into the whites. A rubber spatula is ideal for this job.

Grease a large cookie sheet or spray it with cooking spray.

Spoon heaping tablespoons of the batter one on top of another until you have made 6 rolls. Sprinkle the tops with poppy seeds and bake the rolls for 1 hour. Cool slightly and serve, or store in the refrigerator in a plastic bag.

2.9 grams of carbohydrate in entire recipe; makes 6 rolls, each roll containing 0.5 grams of carbohydrate.

Parmesan Puffs

These make delicious hamburger buns!

Makes 8 puffs

2 extra-large eggs, at room temperature, separated
¼ teaspoon cream of tartar
1 tablespoon cottage cheese
⅛ teaspoon salt
Dash of white pepper
¼ teaspoon ground celery seed
Dash of onion powder
¼ teaspoon baking powder
1 ounce Parmesan cheese, finely grated

Preheat oven to 325° F. Beat egg whites until frothy, add cream of tartar, and continue beating until stiff but not dry. In another bowl, beat egg yolks at high speed with an electric mixer until thick and lemon-yellow. Add cottage cheese, salt, pepper, celery seed, onion powder, and baking powder and beat for another minute. Fold in Parmesan cheese, then gently fold beaten egg whites into yolk-spice mixture. Drop by heaping tablespoonfuls onto a greased cookie sheet and bake for 30 minutes or until golden brown.

2.2 grams of carbohydrate in entire recipe; makes 8 puffs, each containing 0.3 grams of carbohydrate.

Sweet Crêpes

These crêpes are the base for Blintzes (page 53) and Flaming Crêpes (page 54).

Makes 16 crêpes

3 eggs
3 tablespoons fat-free half-and-half
¾ cup cold water
½ teaspoon vanilla extract
1 teaspoon butter extract
Granulated artificial sweetener equal to 3 tablespoons sugar
Pinch of salt
90 grams (¾ cup, unsifted) full-fat soy flour
2 teaspoons whipped butter and 4 teaspoons light olive oil

Combine the eggs, half-and-half, and cold water, vanilla extract, butter extract, artificial sweetener, salt, and soy flour in an electric blender and blend at highest speed for 1 minute. If some flour adheres to sides of blender container, scrape it down with a narrow rubber spatula and blend for 2 to 3 seconds more. Refrigerate the crêpe batter in the covered blender container for 2 hours. When removed from the refrigerator, the batter should be just thick enough to coat a wooden spoon. A tablespoon or 2 of water may be added if batter needs thinning.

With a pastry brush, brush a 6-inch crêpe pan or nonstick skillet with the butter-and-oil mixture. Set over medium-high heat just until the pan begins to smoke. Quickly remove the pan from the flame and pour about 3 tablespoons of the batter right into the middle of the pan. A ¼-cup measuring cup about ¾ filled is convenient for this job. Quickly tilt the pan in all directions to make the batter run all over the bottom of the pan in a thin film. Return the pan to the flame for about 1 minute. Lift crêpe edges with a metal spatula, and if the underside is a nice golden brown, turn the crêpe. Brown the other side for about ½ minute. Slide the crêpe onto aluminum foil or a warm plate. Brush the skillet with fat again, heat just to smoking, and repeat until all batter is used. For suggestions on fillings see *Jam Fillings for Crêpes or Jelly Roll,* page 55.

32 grams of carbohydrate in entire recipe; makes 16 crêpes, each crêpe containing 2.0 grams of carbohydrate.

Sponge Cake Cream Rolls

Butter Sponge Cake Cream Roll

Remember the rich, gooey cakes from your pre-diet days? Well, try this and compare!

Makes 16 slices

30 grams (¼ cup, unsifted) full-fat soy flour
½ teaspoon baking powder
Dash of salt
6 extra-large eggs, at room temperature, separated
¾ teaspoon cream of tartar
1½ teaspoons butter extract
1 teaspoon vanilla extract
5 tablespoons cold water
Granulated artificial sweetener equal to ¾ cup sugar

Preheat oven to 325° F.
 Combine soy flour, baking powder, and salt and set aside. Beat egg whites until foamy, add cream of tartar, and continue beating until stiff but not dry. In another bowl, beat egg yolks at high speed with an electric mixer until thick and lemon-yellow—about 5 minutes. Add extracts, water, and sweetener to egg yolks, and mix until combined. Sift soy flour

mixture into egg yolk mixture and beat until smooth. Gently fold egg yolk mixture into beaten egg whites.

Line a 15½ × 10½ × 1-inch jelly-roll pan with waxed paper and grease with cooking spray or oil. Spread mixture in the prepared pan, and bake for 35 to 40 minutes, or until cake tests done when a cake tester or toothpick is inserted.

Cool cake in the pan for about 5 minutes, then turn it out on a larger sheet of waxed paper. Carefully remove baked-on paper from cake bottom and discard. Roll cake lengthwise, being careful not to break it; use waxed paper as an aid. (Rolling the cake when warm helps to prevent breakage.) When cake is cool, unroll it, and fill with desired Cream Filling. Reroll the cake. Store overnight in the refrigerator in a plastic bag as this improves the texture. This cake combines well with Chocolate Rum Cream Filling, Strawberry Cream Filling, Banana Cream Filling, and Maple Walnut Cream Filling. (See *Cream Fillings for Sponge Cake Cream Rolls,* page 57.)

12.1 grams of carbohydrate in entire recipe without filling; makes 16 slices, each slice containing 0.8 grams of carbohydrate. Add carbohydrates for chosen Cream Filling and divide by 16 to get the count per slice.

NOTE: This cake may also be cut into squares and eaten as a plain sponge cake without filling.

Orange Sponge Cake Cream Roll

Perhaps you prefer orange? Follow ingredients and preparation for Butter Sponge Cake Cream Roll, adding ½ teaspoon orange extract with other extracts. This cake combines well with Orange Brandied Cream Filling (page 60) and with Orange Chocolate Cream Filling (page 61).

Carbohydrate values are the same as for Butter Sponge Cake Cream Roll above.

Yes, You Can Bake with Soy Flour 45

Lemon Sponge Cake Cream Roll

Follow directions for ingredients and preparation for Butter Sponge Cake Cream Roll, adding ½ teaspoon lemon extract with other extracts. This cake combines well with Lemon Butter Cream Filling (page 58).

Carbohydrate values are the same as for Butter Sponge Cake Cream Roll (page 44).

Almond Sponge Cake Cream Roll

Follow directions for ingredients and preparation for Butter Sponge Cake Cream Roll, adding 1 teaspoon almond extract. This cake combines well with Chocolate Almond Cream Filling (page 61).

Carbohydrate values are the same as for Butter Sponge Cake Cream Roll (page 44).

Gingerbread Squares or Spice Cake Cream Roll

How about hot gingerbread with whipped cream?

Makes 18 squares

30 grams (¼ cup, unsifted) full-fat soy flour
½ teaspoon baking powder
Dash of salt
6 extra-large eggs, at room temperature, separated
¾ teaspoon cream of tartar
7 tablespoons cold water
1½ teaspoons nutmeg
1½ teaspoons cloves
1½ teaspoons allspice
1½ teaspoons ginger
1½ teaspoons cinnamon

Granulated artificial sweetener equal to 1¼ cups sugar
½ teaspoon butter extract
½ teaspoon orange extract

To make Gingerbread Squares, follow directions for the preparation of Butter Sponge Cake Cream Roll batter (page 43), adding the spices at the same time as the water and extracts. Bake the cake in a 13 × 9 × 2-inch baking pan for 35 to 40 minutes. When the cake has cooled, cut it in 18 squares. To make half of this recipe, halve the ingredients and bake in an 8-inch square pan. Top the Gingerbread Squares with Vanilla Cream Filling (page 59) or Orange Brandied Cream Filling (page 60).

To make a Spice Sponge Cake Cream Roll, follow the complete preparation instructions for Butter Sponge Cake Cream Roll and bake in a jelly-roll pan. The roll can then be filled with either Vanilla Cream Filling or Orange Brandied Cream Filling.

12.1 grams of carbohydrate in entire recipe. Each slice or piece contains 0.8 grams of carbohydrate.

NOTE: If you halve the Gingerbread Squares recipe, simply halve the carbohydrate count.

Brazil Nut Pie Crust

Try this and see if you don't agree that Brazil nuts make the most delicious pie crust you've ever tasted.

Crust for one 9-inch pie or 6 servings

¼ pound shelled Brazil nuts
Granulated artificial sweetener equal to 2 tablespoons sugar

Chop the Brazil nuts till very fine or grind them in a blender or food processor. Mix the Brazil nuts with the artificial sweetener and press the mixture firmly onto the bottom and sides of a greased 9-inch pie plate. Fill with desired chiffon filling and refrigerate. I like to use a glass pie plate or Corning Ware pie plate, which goes to the table prettily.

12.4 grams of carbohydrate in entire recipe; if serving 6, the crust will contain 2.1 grams per serving.

Sweet Pie Crust (Cookie Crust)

If you want a baked pie crust, try this one.

Makes 6 servings

6 tablespoons sweet butter or trans-fat-free margarine
3 ounces farmer's cheese
Granulated artificial sweetener equal to 2 tablespoons sugar
60 grams (½ cup) full-fat soy flour, sifted
An additional 15 grams of soy flour

Preheat oven to 350° F. Cream together butter and farmer's cheese with an electric mixer or blender. Mix in artificial sweetener. Gradually add soy flour and combine thoroughly. Wrap dough in waxed paper or plastic wrap and chill in refrigerator for 1 to 2 hours until dough is firm enough to roll.

The easiest way to roll this dough is between sheets of waxed paper, remembering to loosen both the upper and lower papers several times to prevent sticking. Place 1 sheet of waxed paper on a firm, flat surface, sift a little of the extra 15 grams of soy flour all over paper, and place ball of dough on top. Sift a bit more of remaining soy flour on top of the dough and place a second sheet of waxed paper on top. Roll dough to fit a 9-inch pie pan and invert it over the pan. Work fast. If dough should tear a little, do not reroll. (This dough may be patched.) I like to flute the edges by placing 1 finger between 2 fingers of the opposite hand and pressing the resulting design around the entire edge. This takes just a few extra minutes and looks so much prettier.

Bake the crust in the preheated oven for 12 to 14 minutes before using. This crust may also be baked with filling in it. Follow filling recipe directions.

25.0 grams of carbohydrate in entire pie crust; if serving 6, the crust for each serving contains 4.2 grams of carbohydrate.

II.

The Sweet Things in Life

Brandy Nut Kisses　　51
Jam Sandwich Cookies　　52
Blintzes　　53
Flaming Crêpes　　54
Jelly Roll　　55
Jam Fillings for Crêpes or Jelly Roll　　55
Cream Fillings for Sponge Cake Cream Rolls　　57
Strawberry Shortcake　　62
Individual Strawberry Shortcakes　　63
Cheesecakes　　64
Rhubarb Sauce or Stewed Rhubarb　　69
Dessert Omelets　　70
Dessert Soufflés　　73
Puddings and Pie Fillings　　76
Chocolate Mousse　　80
Lemon Mousse　　81
Tiramisu　　82
Berry Misu　　84
Ice Creams　　85
Granites　　89
Zabaglione　　91
Frio, Frio　　92
Ice Pops　　92
Some Sweet Diet Drinks　　93

The Sweet Things in Life

I have deliberately put my dessert chapter at the front of my book because I have found that sweets are what dieters seem to miss most. On many diets, including most low-carbohydrate diets, you can eat interesting appetizers, delicious main courses, tasty salads and vegetables, fine Continental foods, but *no* fancy desserts. This chapter gives a multitude of tasty desserts back to you—with a minimum of carbohydrates. Enjoy them and use them to lose weight as well as to stay thin.

Brandy Nut Kisses

Makes 24 cookies

3 egg whites, at room temperature
Pinch of salt
½ teaspoon cream of tartar
1 teaspoon Cognac
Granulated artificial sweetener equal to ¾ cup sugar
1 cup very finely chopped pecans

Preheat oven to 250° F. Beat egg whites until foamy, add salt and cream of tartar, and continue beating until stiff but not dry. Add Cognac and artificial sweetener and beat 1 minute more. Very gently fold in pecans. Drop by teaspoonfuls onto a greased cookie sheet and bake approximately 30 to 35 minutes or until dry. When cooled, store cookies in an airtight container.

16.8 grams of carbohydrate in entire recipe; makes 24 kisses, each cookie containing 0.7 grams of carbohydrate.

Jam Sandwich Cookies

Makes 12 cookies

2 extra-large eggs
Granulated artificial sweetener equal to 3 tablespoons sugar
¼ teaspoon butter extract
½ teaspoon lemon extract
¼ teaspoon vanilla
1 teaspoon cold water
Cooking spray
2 ounces diet apricot jam

Preheat oven to 325° F. Beat eggs with an electric mixer at high speed until the eggs become very thick and lemon-colored. This should take at least 10 minutes. Mix in artificial sweetener, extracts, and water.

Grease muffin pans with cooking spray (for 24) and divide mixture among the 24 spaces. Bake 10 minutes. Remove pans from oven and cool cookies.

When cookies have cooled, spread 12 of the cookies with diet apricot jam, using about 2 ounces in all. Cover these 12 cookies with the remaining 12 cookies, forming sandwich cookies. Store in the refrigerator in a plastic bag.

2.0 grams of carbohydrate in entire recipe; makes 12 cookies, each cookie containing 0.2 grams of carbohydrate.

Blintzes

Years ago whenever I went to the old Lindy's, blintzes were my favorite dish.

Makes 16 blintzes

1 recipe Sweet Crêpes (page 42)
1 egg
2 ounces cream cheese, softened (or Neufchatel, ⅓ less fat than cream cheese)
6 ounces farmer's cheese, softened
Granulated artificial sweetener equal to 3 tablespoons sugar
Dash of cinnamon
Scant ½ teaspoon vanilla extract
2 teaspoons whipped butter and 1 tablespoon light olive oil
Sour cream, 50 percent reduced fat
Sugarless strawberry jam

Prepare crêpe batter and refrigerate at least 2 hours in advance. Cook crêpes just before making the filling for blintzes and keep warm.

Mix together in an electric mixer until smooth the egg, cream cheese, farmer's cheese, artificial sweetener, cinnamon, and vanilla. Put about 1 rounded teaspoonful of cheese mixture in the center of each sweet crêpe and roll it up, folding in the sides to make a little sealed package. Repeat until all cheese mixture and blintzes have been used. Melt 1 tablespoon butter mixture in a large skillet and sauté the blintzes until golden brown. Add remaining butter mixture, turn blintzes, and brown on other side. Serve hot with sour cream and sugarless strawberry jam.

35.6 grams of carbohydrate in entire recipe; makes 16 blintzes, each blintz containing 2.2 grams of carbohydrate. Add 1.5 grams of carbohydrate for each table-

spoon of sour cream used. Check jam jar for carbohydrate content as brands and flavors vary.

Flaming Crêpes

Crêpes make an impressive dessert for company. Just don't set the house on fire when you flame them.

Makes 8 servings

1 recipe Sweet Crêpes (page 42)
2 jars any Jam Fillings for Crêpes or Jelly Roll (page 55)
4 teaspoons melted whipped butter and 2 tablespoons very light olive oil
4 tablespoons kirsch, Grand Marnier, or peach or apricot brandy
Additional granulated artificial sweetener

Prepare crêpe batter and refrigerate at least 2 hours in advance. Make and fill crêpes before guests arrive. Lay each crêpe on a flat surface. Place 2 teaspoons of Jam Filling in the center, roll up, and place in a shallow baking dish. When all crêpes are filled, sprinkle with the melted butter and oil mixture.

Just before serving, place the dish in a preheated 350° F. oven for 5 to 10 minutes to warm the crêpes. Warm the brandy or liqueur slightly. Pour warmed spirits over crêpes and ignite with a long fireplace match or a kitchen match. When flames die down, sprinkle on a little extra granulated artificial sweetener. Serve hot.

If made with kirsch, 40.8 grams of carbohydrate in entire recipe; if serving 8, each serving contains 5.1 grams of carbohydrate (plus carbohydrate from Jam Filling).
If using Grand Marnier or peach or apricot brandy, 43.2 grams of carbohydrate in entire recipe; if serving 8, each serving contains 5.4 grams of carbohydrate (plus carbohydrate from Jam Filling).

Jelly Roll

A dietetic version of an old-fashioned jelly roll.

Makes 16 slices of cake

1 recipe for Butter Sponge Cake Cream Roll (page 43) or
  Almond Sponge Cake Cream Roll (page 45)
2 cups any Jam Filling for Crêpes or Jelly Roll (below)

When cake has cooled completely, spread with jam filling, using a metal spatula. Roll the cake and place on an attractive serving dish. Refrigerate until serving time, then cut it in 16 slices.

If using Jam Filling made with kirsch, 20.1 grams of carbohydrate in entire recipe (with other liqueurs, 34.5 grams); makes 16 slices of cake, each slice containing 1.3 grams of carbohydrate (with other liqueurs, 2.2 grams).

Jam Fillings for Crêpes or Jelly Roll

Apricot Jam Filling

Grand Marnier is marvelous when mixed with apricot.

Makes 1 cup

1 cup (8 ounces) sugarless apricot jam
1 tablespoon Grand Marnier or apricot brandy
Granulated artificial sweetener equal to ½ cup sugar

Mix all ingredients together thoroughly. This filling may be made in advance and stored in the refrigerator until needed.

83.5 grams of carbohydrate in entire recipe, each teaspoonful containing 1.7 grams of carbohydrate.

Cherry or Blackberry Jam Filling

Makes 1 cup

1 cup (8 ounces) sugarless cherry jam or sugarless blackberry jam
2 teaspoons kirsch
Granulated artificial sweetener equal to ¼ cup sugar

Mix all ingredients together thoroughly. This filling may be made in advance and stored in the refrigerator until needed. I generally just return it to the jam jar.

82.0 grams of carbohydrate in entire recipe, each teaspoonful containing 1.7 grams of carbohydrate.

Raspberry Jam Filling

Makes 1 cup

1 cup (8 ounces) sugarless raspberry jam
2 teaspoons kirsch
Granulated artificial sweetener equal to 3 tablespoons sugar

Mix all ingredients together thoroughly. Store in the refrigerator until needed.

Carbohydrate values are the same as for Cherry Jam Filling.

Strawberry Jam Filling

Makes 1 cup

1 cup (8 ounces) sugarless strawberry jam
1 teaspoon kirsch

Granulated artificial sweetener equal to 10 tablespoons sugar

Mix all ingredients together thoroughly. Store in the refrigerator to use as needed.

81.0 grams of carbohydrate in entire recipe, each teaspoonful containing 1.7 grams of carbohydrate.

Cream Fillings for Sponge Cake Cream Rolls

Banana Cream Filling

Filling for 16 slices of cake

12 ounces ricotta cheese, part-skim variety
2 teaspoons banana extract
½ teaspoon vanilla extract
1 teaspoon fresh lemon juice
Artificial sweetener equal to ¼ cup sugar

Beat ricotta cheese with electric mixer until smooth and creamy. Add banana extract, vanilla extract, lemon juice, and sweetener and beat until well combined. Refrigerate until cake has finished baking and cooling. This filling combines well with Butter Sponge Cake Cream Roll (page 43).

16.0 grams of carbohydrate in entire recipe; when used as a filling for 16 slices of cake, the filling will contain 1.0 grams per slice.

58 THE LOW-CARB GOURMET

Lemon Butter Cream Filling

Filling for 16 slices of cake

12 ounces ricotta cheese, part-skim variety
1 teaspoon fresh lemon juice
¼ teaspoon vanilla extract
¾ teaspoon lemon extract
¼ teaspoon butter extract
½ teaspoon freshly grated lemon peel
¼ teaspoon ground mace
Artificial sweetener equal to ¼ cup sugar

Follow directions for Banana Cream Filling (page 57).

Carbohydrate values are the same as for Banana Cream Filling.

Maple Walnut Cream Filling

Filling for 16 slices of cake

12 ounces ricotta cheese, part-skim variety
1 teaspoon maple extract
20 drops vanilla extract
Artificial sweetener equal to 6 tablespoons sugar
2½ ounces coarsely chopped walnuts (about ½ cup plus 2 tablespoons)

Follow directions for Banana Cream Filling (page 57), folding in the chopped walnuts at the very end.

26.9 grams of carbohydrate in entire recipe; when used as filling for 16 slices of cake, the filling will contain 1.7 grams per slice.

The Sweet Things in Life 59

Strawberry Cream Filling

Filling for 16 slices of cake

12 ounces ricotta cheese, part-skim variety
1 teaspoon vanilla extract
Artificial sweetener equal to 6 tablespoons sugar
1 cup fresh strawberries, sliced

Follow directions for Banana Cream Filling (page 57), folding in the strawberries at the very end.

28.8 grams of carbohydrate in entire recipe; when used as filling for 16 slices of cake, the filling will contain 1.8 grams per slice.

Vanilla Cream Filling

Filling for 16 slices of cake

12 ounces ricotta cheese, part-skim variety
1 scant teaspoon vanilla extract
Artificial sweetener equal to 6 tablespoons sugar

Follow directions for Banana Cream Filling (page 57).

16.0 grams of carbohydrate in entire recipe; when used as filling for 16 slices of cake, the filling will contain 1.0 grams per slice.

NOTE: Try topping your hot gingerbread with this instead of whipped cream.

Orange Brandied Cream Filling

Filling for 16 slices of cake

12 ounces ricotta cheese, part-skim variety
1¼ teaspoons orange extract
1¼ teaspoons Cognac
¼ teaspoon butter extract
Artificial sweetener equal to 6 tablespoons sugar
3 drops red food coloring
9 drops yellow food coloring

Follow directions for Banana Cream Filling (page 57). This filling combines well with Orange Sponge Cake Cream Roll (page 44).

16.0 grams of carbohydrate in entire recipe; when used as a filling for 16 slices of cake, the filling will contain 1.0 grams per slice.

Chocolate Rum Cream Filling

Filling for 16 slices of cake

12 ounces ricotta cheese, part-skim variety
1 square unsweetened chocolate, melted
4 teaspoons chocolate extract
10 drops mocha extract
½ teaspoon rum extract
1 tablespoon dark rum
Artificial sweetener equal to ½ cup sugar

Beat ricotta cheese with electric mixer until smooth and creamy. Melt chocolate and beat in immediately. Add extracts, rum, and sweetener and beat till well combined. Refrigerate until cake has finished baking and cooling. This filling combines well with Butter Sponge Cake Cream Roll (page 43).

24.0 grams of carbohydrate in entire recipe; when used as filling for 16 slices of cake, the filling will contain 1.5 grams per slice.

NOTE: This may also be served in dessert dishes such as Chocolate Rum Ricotta Mousse.

Orange Chocolate Cream Filling

Filling for 16 slices of cake

12 ounces ricotta cheese, part-skim variety
1 square unsweetened chocolate, melted
4 teaspoons chocolate extract
½ teaspoon orange extract
1 teaspoon Cognac
Artificial sweetener equal to ½ cup sugar

Follow directions for Chocolate Rum Cream Filling (page 60).

Carbohydrate values are the same as for Chocolate Rum Cream Filling.

Chocolate Almond Cream Filling

Filling for 16 slices of cake

12 ounces ricotta cheese, part-skim variety
1 square unsweetened chocolate, melted
5 teaspoons chocolate extract
½ teaspoon almond extract
½ teaspoon vanilla extract
Scant ¼ teaspoon mocha extract
Artificial sweetener equal to ½ cup sugar

Follow directions for Chocolate Rum Cream Filling (page 60). This filling combines well with Almond Sponge Cake Cream Roll (page 45).

62   THE LOW-CARB GOURMET

24.0 grams of carbohydrate in entire recipe; when used as filling for 16 slices of cake, the filling will contain 1.5 grams per slice.

Strawberry Shortcake

An old favorite in a new dietetic version.

Makes 8 servings

1 recipe Butter Sponge Cake (page 43) or Almond Butter Sponge Cake (page 45)
300 grams (about 10½ ounces) fresh strawberries
1 recipe Vanilla Cream Filling (page 59)
Nonstick cooking spray

Preheat oven to 325° F. and line the bottoms of two 9-inch layer cake pans with waxed paper. (Trace the pan outline with a sharp instrument like a pair of scissors, then cut out the waxed paper circle.) Grease the pans, paper and all, with cooking spray.

Prepare batter for sponge cake and divide equally between the 2 pans. Bake in preheated oven 35 minutes.

When the cakes are done, cool 10 minutes, then unmold from the pan, removing the waxed paper, and cool completely. Baking may be done earlier in the day. Then, wrap the cake in aluminum foil after cooling and refrigerate until ready to serve.

Wash and hull the strawberries. Set aside the 7 largest and most beautiful for decorating the top of the cake. Slice remaining berries. Prepare Vanilla Cream Filling or another flavor of your choice (pages 55–61).

Spread approximately a third of this mixture on 1 layer of cake. Add the sliced strawberries, combining them with the cream. Top with the second layer of cake. Spread the remaining cream mixture first on the sides and then on the top of the cake. Decorate with the whole strawberries.

Refrigerate carefully until serving time.

43.2 grams of carbohydrate in entire recipe; if serving 8, each serving contains 5.4 grams of carbohydrate.

Individual Strawberry Shortcakes

Makes 4 servings

4 Easy-Mix Muffins (page 31)
400 grams fresh strawberries (about 14 ounces)
4 teaspoons Cognac
20 drops orange extract (¼ teaspoon)
Granulated artificial sweetener equal to ¼ cup sugar
1 recipe Vanilla Cream Filling (page 59)

Slice each muffin in half. Reserve 12 of the prettiest whole strawberries. Mash remaining strawberries and add the Cognac, orange extract, and artificial sweetener. Mix thoroughly and set aside.

Place a muffin half in each of 4 dishes. Top with a generous scoop of the cream mixture, then top cream with some mashed strawberries, dividing the berries evenly among the 4 portions. Blend the strawberries into the cream slightly by moving a teaspoon around each. Top each with the other muffin half. Spoon remaining cream over all 4 portions. Decorate with 3 whole strawberries on top of each shortcake, and refrigerate until serving time.

51.2 grams of carbohydrate in entire recipe; if serving 4, each serving contains 12.8 grams of carbohydrate.

NOTE: These strawberry shortcakes are a little higher in carbohydrates than some of my other desserts, but if you have muffins in the house as I always do, they can be made in an emergency when you have nothing else for dessert that is nonfattening. Great for unexpected company, which is the origin of this recipe, and actually it's the fruit that provides most of the carbohydrates.

Cheesecakes

Cheesecake Supreme

Makes 12 servings

6 extra-large eggs, at room temperature, separated
2 teaspoons vanilla extract
1 teaspoon fresh lemon juice
¼ teaspoon ground cinnamon
½ teaspoon fresh orange peel
½ teaspoon fresh lemon peel
Granulated artificial sweetener equal to 1¼ cups sugar
½ pound Neufchâtel cheese (⅓ less fat than cream cheese)
1½ pounds farmer's cheese
¾ teaspoon cream of tartar

Preheat oven to 325° F. In a blender or food processor combine egg yolks, vanilla, lemon juice, cinnamon, orange peel, lemon peel, and artificial sweetener and blend thoroughly. Add Neufchâtel cheese to blender a third at a time and blend thoroughly after each addition. Add the farmer's cheese gradually in the same way and continue to blend until smooth.

This is a very thick mixture and should be blended at the highest speed. When half the farmer's cheese has been added and the action slows, stop the blender and use a slim rubber spatula to push the ingredients from the container sides and to stir up from the bottom. Be sure to turn the motor off before using the rubber spatula.

Beat egg whites until foamy, add cream of tartar, and continue beating until stiff but not dry. Gently fold the cheese mixture into the beaten whites.

Grease a 2½-quart baking dish or springform pan and fill with cheesecake mixture. Bake at 325° F. 15 minutes, then raise temperature to 425° F. and continue baking another 8 minutes. Turn off the oven, leaving the cake in it.

Gradually open the oven door, a little at a time. Open a little more every 5 or 10 minutes until the oven door is completely open. The cake should sit in the oven for about 1 hour after the oven has been turned off. To improve both the taste and the texture of the cake, refrigerate overnight.

30.1 grams of carbohydrate in entire recipe; if serving 12, each serving contains 2.5 grams of carbohydrate.

Marble Cheesecake

Makes 10 servings

Cheesecake Batter

6 eggs
2 tablespoons lemon juice
2 teaspoons vanilla extract
4 teaspoons peanut oil
Granulated artificial sweetener equal to 1 cup sugar
2 pounds very dry pot cheese

Marble Mixture

½ cup cheesecake batter
Granulated artificial sweetener equal to 1½ cups sugar
1 teaspoon vanilla extract
2 tablespoons chocolate extract
1 ounce (1 square) unsweetened chocolate, melted
Food coloring, if desired

Preheat oven to 350° F. Have all ingredients at room temperature. In a blender, combine eggs, lemon juice, vanilla, oil, and artificial sweetener and blend thoroughly. Add pot cheese gradually and continue to blend until very smooth. Grease a 9 × 5 × 3-inch loaf pan and pour batter into it, reserving ½ cup batter in the blender container.

To make the marble mixture, add to reserved cheesecake batter the artificial sweetener, extracts, and melted chocolate and blend until combined. Add food coloring, if desired, to deepen the chocolate color. Gently drop spoonfuls of marble mixture on cheesecake batter in the prepared pan. Cut through batter with a knife or metal spatula several times for a marbled effect. Bake 40 minutes or until cake is firm. Turn off the oven, leaving the cake in it.

Gradually open the oven door, a little at a time, every 5 or 10 minutes until door is completely open. Cake should sit in the oven for about 1 to 1½ hours from the time the oven is turned off. Chill cake overnight to develop the flavor. The cake will settle as it cools.

29 grams of carbohydrate in entire recipe; if serving 10, each serving contains 2.9 grams of carbohydrate.

Refrigerator Italian Cheesecake

My version of an Italian Cheesecake that doesn't need to be baked.

Makes 10 servings

1 envelope unflavored gelatin
½ cup cold water
3 tablespoons fat-free half-and-half
1 extra-large egg, at room temperature, separated
Dash of salt
1 pound ricotta cheese, part-skim variety
1 teaspoon vanilla extract
½ teaspoon almond extract

½ teaspoon freshly grated lemon peel
Granulated artificial sweetener equal to ½ cup plus
   2 tablespoons sugar
⅛ teaspoon cream of tartar

Soften gelatin cold water for 5 minutes in the top of a double boiler. Add half-and-half, egg yolk, and salt and heat, stirring frequently with a wire whisk, until the mixture thickens. (Do not allow to boil.) Cool the mixture slightly and empty it into a blender. Add the ricotta, vanilla and almond extracts, lemon peel, and artificial sweetener and blend until smooth and well combined. Beat egg white till foamy, add cream of tartar, and continue beating until stiff but not dry. Fold in the ricotta mixture. Place the batter in a 9 × 5 × 3-inch glass or a Corning Ware loaf pan and refrigerate until firm.

24.2 grams of carbohydrate in entire recipe; if serving 10, each serving contains 2.4 grams of carbohydrate.

Refrigerator Banana Cheesecake

Makes 8 servings

2 envelopes unflavored gelatin
1¼ cups water
2 extra-large eggs, at room temperature, separated
¼ teaspoon salt
2 tablespoons lemon juice
Granulated artificial sweetener equal to 2 cups sugar
4 teaspoons banana extract
½ teaspoon vanilla extract
½ teaspoon almond extract
24 ounces (1½ pounds) reduced fat cottage cheese
¼ teaspoon cream of tartar

Put gelatin into blender or food processor with ½ cup cold water and stir to dissolve gelatin. Combine remaining water, egg yolks, salt, and lemon juice in the top of a double boiler and heat, stirring frequently, until slightly thickened. Remove from stove and add to blender. Add artificial sweetener and extracts and stir again. Raise blender speed higher, and add cottage cheese, about 8 ounces at a time, and blend until smooth, but not watery.

Beat egg whites until foamy, add cream of tartar, and continue beating until stiff but not dry. Gently fold beaten egg whites into cheese mixture. Butter a cake pan or a mold, then rinse with ice cold water. Shake out any excess water, but do not dry it. Empty cheesecake mixture into prepared pan and refrigerate until firm. To serve, unmold onto a serving dish and garnish with fresh strawberries.

20.2 grams of carbohydrate in entire recipe; if serving 8, each serving contains 2.5 grams of carbohydrate.

Refrigerator Lemon Cheesecake

Makes 8 servings

2 envelopes unflavored gelatin
1¼ cups cold water
2 extra-large eggs, at room temperature, separated
¼ teaspoon salt
2 tablespoons lemon juice
Artificial sweetener equal to 2½ cups sugar
1 teaspoon vanilla extract
½ teaspoon lemon extract
2 teaspoons freshly grated lemon peel
1 teaspoon freshly grated orange peel
24 ounces (1½ pounds) cottage cheese
¼ teaspoon cream of tartar

Follow directions for Refrigerator Banana Cheesecake (above), adding lemon peel and orange peel to the blender along with the extracts.

20.2 grams of carbohydrate in entire recipe; if serving 8, each serving contains 2.5 grams of carbohydrate.

Rhubarb Sauce or Stewed Rhubarb

Makes 5 servings

3 pounds fresh rhubarb
½ cup water
1 tablespoon plus ½ teaspoon fresh lemon juice
¼–½ teaspoon cinnamon
1½ teaspoons vanilla extract
Artificial sweetener equal to 1 cup plus 2 tablespoons sugar

Wash rhubarb, trim, and cut in 1-inch pieces. Pull off any skin that is too tough to cut, stripping it down the length of the stalk. Place in a saucepan over very low heat. Add the water, lemon juice, and cinnamon; cover, and cook gently until tender and juicy, about 20 to 25 minutes. Remove from heat and add vanilla and artificial sweetener. Cool slightly, then place in a blender and purée 1 or 2 minutes until it becomes smooth sauce. This can be eaten either warm or cold.

24.2 grams of carbohydrate in entire recipe; if serving 5, each serving contains 4.8 grams of carbohydrate.

NOTE: If you prefer a more roughly textured rhubarb sauce, omit the blending.

Dessert Omelets

Before making any of these omelets, see General Directions for Omelet Making, page 177.

Sweet Puffy Omelet

A delicate, elegant, sweet omelet.

Makes 1 or 2 servings

2 extra-large eggs, at room temperature, separated
Artificial sweetener equal to 1 teaspoon sugar
¼ teaspoon vanilla extract
1 teaspoon whipped butter and 2 teaspoons very light olive oil
Additional granulated artificial sweetener for sprinkling on top

Beat egg whites until stiff but not dry. Add sweetener and vanilla to egg yolks and beat until thickened. Very gently, with a rubber spatula, fold yolk mixture into beaten egg whites.

Melt butter and oil over high heat in a 10-inch treated or nonstick omelet pan. When butter begins to brown slightly, pour in egg mixture and smooth it out evenly to the pan edges. Reduce heat to moderately low. When the bottom of the omelet is golden brown (lift edges with spatula to see) and the top somewhat puffy, turn omelet out onto a warmed platter. To do this, slide omelet halfway onto platter, then fold remaining half over it. Sprinkle top generously with powdered sweetener and serve immediately. Sweetener mixed with cinnamon would also be good.

1.0 grams of carbohydrate in entire recipe; if serving 2, each portion contains 0.5 grams of carbohydrate.

The Sweet Things in Life

NOTE: Before folding the omelet over, you may spread the top with a sugarless jam, or you can serve some sugarless jam along with the omelet.

Sweet Puffy Almond Omelet

Makes 1 or 2 servings

2 extra-large eggs, at room temperature, separated
15 drops almond extract
Granulated artificial sweetener equal to 2 teaspoons sugar
1 teaspoon whipped butter and 2 teaspoons very light olive oil
Additional granulated artificial sweetener to sprinkle on top
1 tablespoon slivered, toasted almonds

Follow directions for Sweet Puffy Omelet (page 70), adding the almond extract to the egg yolks. Sprinkle the finished omelet with the toasted almonds before sprinkling with the sweetener.

2.5 grams of carbohydrate in entire recipe; if serving 2, each serving contains 1.3 grams of carbohydrate.

Sweet Puffy Lemon Omelet

Makes 1 or 2 servings

2 extra-large eggs, at room temperature, separated
15 drops lemon extract
1 teaspoon fresh lemon juice
1 teaspoon freshly grated lemon peel
Granulated artificial sweetener equal to 2 teaspoons sugar
1 teaspoon whipped butter and 2 teaspoons very light olive oil
Additional granulated artificial sweetener to sprinkle on top

Follow directions for Sweet Puffy Omelet (page 70), adding the lemon peel, lemon juice, extract, and artificial sweetener to the egg yolks. Turn out omelet and sprinkle with granulated sweetener.

1.4 grams of carbohydrate in entire recipe; if serving 2, each portion contains 0.7 grams of carbohydrate.

Strawberry Dessert Omelet

Looking for something unusual to serve for Saturday or Sunday brunch?

Makes 2 servings

1 cup coarsely chopped fresh strawberries
Granulated artificial sweetener equal to 3 tablespoons sugar
1 tablespoon artificially sweetened diet apricot jam, melted
2 extra-large eggs, at room temperature, separated
¼ teaspoon cream of tartar
⅛ teaspoon vanilla extract
Dash of salt
1 teaspoon whipped butter and 2 teaspoons very light olive oil
2 whole strawberries for garnish

Combine chopped strawberries and 1 tablespoon artificial sweetener and set aside. Combine melted jam and 1 tablespoon artificial sweetener and set aside.

Beat egg whites with cream of tartar until stiff but not dry. Without washing beater, beat egg yolks till they are thick and lemon-colored. Add vanilla, remaining 1 tablespoon artificial sweetener, and salt and beat thoroughly. Gently fold beaten egg whites into beaten yolks.

Melt the butter and oil in a hot omelet pan, turning to coat bottom and sides of pan. Pour in eggs. Lower heat and cook omelet until golden brown on the bottom and well puffed up. Spread the chopped strawberries over half the omelet, fold over remaining half, and turn out onto a warm platter. Top with the melted jam and garnish with whole strawberries.

14.0 grams of carbohydrate in entire recipe; if serving 2, each serving contains 7.0 grams of carbohydrate.

NOTE: Strawberry jam or orange marmalade are nice with this, too. Use same amount of sweetener as when using the apricot jam.

Dessert Soufflés

Chocolate Berry Soufflé

Makes 2 servings

2 extra-large eggs, at room temperature, separated
¼ teaspoon cream of tartar
Granulated artificial sweetener equal to 2 tablespoons sugar
2 teaspoons unsweetened Dutch cocoa
2 teaspoons artificially sweetened raspberry preserves*
Artificial sweetener equal to 1 teaspoon sugar

Preheat oven to 375° F. Grease either a 7-inch frying pan, a 1½-cup au gratin dish, or a 1½-cup soufflé dish.

Beat egg whites until foamy, add cream of tartar, and continue beating until stiff but not dry. Beat egg yolks lightly with artificial sweetener equal to 2 tablespoons of sugar, and cocoa. Mix preserves with artificial sweetener equal to 1 teaspoon sugar and spoon preserves into bottom of dish. Top with chocolate egg mixture.

Bake in preheated oven 12 to 14 minutes, or until the soufflé is well puffed. Serve immediately as this soufflé falls quickly.

*If sugar-free cherry preserves are not available, substitute raspberry or strawberry preserves.

4.5 grams of carbohydrate in entire recipe; if serving 2, each serving contains 2.3 grams of carbohydrate.

Lovely Lemon Soufflé

Makes 4 servings

4 extra-large eggs, at room temperature, separated
1 extra egg white, at room temperature
½ teaspoon cream of tartar
Granulated artificial sweetener equal to ½ cup sugar
3 tablespoons fresh lemon juice
1 tablespoon freshly grated lemon peel

Preheat oven to 400° F. Beat all 5 egg whites until foamy, add cream of tartar, and continue beating until stiff but not dry. Without washing beater, beat egg yolks until thick and lemon-colored. Gradually add artificial sweetener while beating the yolks, then beat in lemon juice and lemon peel. Blend a fourth of the egg whites into the egg yolk mixture, then very gently fold in remaining whites.

Pour mixture into a greased 1-quart soufflé dish on which you have put a waxed-paper collar. Bake for 15 to 20 minutes, depending on the degree of firmness you desire. The soufflé should be puffy and high, firm on the outside, and slightly runny inside. The longer baking time will yield a firmer soufflé.

5.6 grams of carbohydrate in entire recipe; if serving 4, each serving contains 1.4 grams of carbohydrate.

The Sweet Things in Life

Frozen Pumpkin Soufflé

Why not try this pumpkin soufflé instead of pumpkin pie?

Makes 6 servings

1 envelope unflavored gelatin
¼ cup dark rum
4 extra-large eggs, at room temperature
Granulated artificial sweetener equal to ⅔ cup sugar
1 cup pumpkin, home-cooked or canned
½ teaspoon cinnamon
½ teaspoon ginger
¼ teaspoon mace
¼ teaspoon cloves
½ cup fat-free half-and-half
1 extra egg white, at room temperature
⅛ teaspoon cream of tartar

Prepare a 6-inch waxed paper or aluminum foil collar on a 1-quart soufflé dish and set aside.

In a saucepan, soften 1 envelope gelatin in ¼ cup dark rum for 5 minutes. Heat gelatin over simmering water or over gentle heat until dissolved and set aside. Beat the 4 eggs thoroughly, add artificial sweetener, and continue beating until mixture is very thick. Mix together the pumpkin, cinnamon, ginger, mace, and cloves, then add the gelatin-rum mixture to the flavored pumpkin. Mix together thoroughly. Mix in the half-and-half thoroughly.

Beat the egg white until foamy, add the cream of tartar, and continue beating until stiff but not dry. Very gently fold beaten egg white into pumpkin mixture.

Turn soufflé into prepared dish and chill until firmly set. Remove the paper collar carefully before serving.

33.5 grams of carbohydrate in entire recipe; if serving 6, each serving contains 5.6 grams of carbohydrate.

Puddings and Pie Fillings

Chocolate Almond Pie Filling or Pudding

Filling for one 9-inch pie or 6 servings

1 envelope unflavored gelatin
½ cup fat-free half-and-half
1½ cups cold water
1 square unsweetened chocolate, melted
3 extra-large eggs, at room temperature, separated
1 teaspoon vanilla extract
½ teaspoon almond extract
Artificial sweetener equal to 1 cup sugar
¼ teaspoon cream of tartar

Soften gelatin in the half-and-half. Boil water and add to gelatin mixture, stirring to dissolve gelatin. Mix in melted chocolate. Beat in egg yolks, 1 at a time, beating thoroughly after each addition. Place mixture in top of a double boiler or over gentle heat and cook, stirring constantly until thickened. Remove from heat and blend in extracts and artificial sweetener.

Beat egg whites until frothy, add cream of tartar, and continue beating until stiff but not dry. Gently fold beaten egg whites into chocolate mixture and turn into a pie shell or into decorative dessert dishes. Refrigerate until serving time.

17.1 grams of carbohydrate in entire recipe; if serving 6, the filling will contain 2.9 grams per serving.

Lemon Chiffon Pie Filling or Pudding

The combination of lemon chiffon with Brazil nuts is unbelievable.

Filling for one 9-inch pie or 6 servings

1 envelope unflavored gelatin
¼ cup cold water
½ cup fresh lemon juice
Dash of salt
1–2 teaspoons freshly grated lemon peel, as desired
4 extra-large eggs, at room temperature, separated
Granulated artificial sweetener equal to 1½ cups sugar
½ teaspoon cream of tartar

Soften gelatin in cold water. In the top of a double boiler or in a heavy pot placed over gentle heat, combine lemon juice, salt, and lemon rind. Beat in the egg yolks, 1 at a time, then cook, stirring constantly, until mixture thickens and coats a spoon (it must not boil). Stir in softened gelatin. Remove from heat and add artificial sweetener.

Beat egg whites until foamy, add cream of tartar, and continue beating until stiff but not dry. Fold egg whites gently into the lemon custard. Turn into pie shell or pretty dessert dishes and chill.

Refrigerate until serving time.

11.9 grams of carbohydrate in entire recipe; if serving 6, the filling will contain 2.0 grams per serving.

Lime Chiffon Pie Filling or Pudding

Filling for one 9-inch pie or 6 servings

Follow recipe for Lemon Chiffon Pie Filling, above, substituting ½ cup fresh lime juice for the fresh lemon juice, and substituting 2 teaspoons freshly grated lime peel for the grated lemon peel.

13.0 grams of carbohydrate in entire recipe; if serving 6, the filling will contain 2.2 grams per serving.

NOTE: Both Lemon Chiffon and Lime Chiffon Pie Fillings make a nice frozen soufflé also. Prepare the soufflé dish with

78 THE LOW-CARB GOURMET

a waxed-paper collar. Then before bringing the soufflé to the table, remove the collar.

Lemon Cake-Pudding

Makes 6 servings

5 extra-large eggs
Granulated artificial sweetener equal to 1 cup sugar
3 tablespoons fresh lemon juice
Grated peel from 1 fresh lemon

Preheat oven to 325° F. Beat the eggs at high speed with an electric mixer until very thick and lemon-colored. Add the sweetener and continue beating a few more minutes. Stir in, at lowest speed of the mixer, the lemon juice and lemon peel. Pour mixture into a 2-quart ovenproof soufflé dish. Set this dish into a larger pan containing 1 to 1½ inches of hot water. Bake the cake-pudding 30 minutes. Refrigerate until serving time.

6.1 grams of carbohydrate in entire recipe; if serving 6, each serving contains 1.0 gram each.

Lemon Pudding

This dessert can be used for even the strictest versions of the low-carbohydrate diet. You don't have to feel deprived at all now.

Makes 5 servings

1 envelope unflavored gelatin
¼ cup cold water
1½ cups boiling water
2 extra-large eggs, at room temperature, separated
Dash of salt
Granulated artificial sweetener equal to ¼ cup sugar

¼ cup lemon juice
1 teaspoon vanilla extract
Grated peel of 1 lemon
¼ teaspoon mace
¼ teaspoon cream of tartar

Soften gelatin in cold water. Add boiling water and stir until gelatin is dissolved. Pour gelatin mixture into top of a double boiler or into a heavy saucepan over gentle heat. Beat in the egg yolks, then add salt, and heat until mixture thickens. Remove from heat and add artificial sweetener, lemon juice, vanilla, lemon peel, and mace. Chill in refrigerator until mixture becomes syrupy.

Beat egg whites until frothy, add cream of tartar, and continue beating until stiff but not dry. Gently fold egg whites into lemon mixture. Rinse out a 3½–4-cup mold with icy cold water and fill with lemon pudding. Refrigerate until firm. Unmold to serve, and garnish with fresh strawberries.

5.8 grams of carbohydrate in entire recipe; if serving 5, each serving contains 1.2 grams of carbohydrate.

Raspberry Sponge Pudding

This delightful, fresh-tasting pudding has hardly any carbohydrates or calories.

Makes 6 servings

1 envelope unflavored gelatin
½ cup cold water
1 cup fresh raspberries
1 cup boiling water
1½ teaspoons fresh lemon juice
Artificial sweetener equal to ½ cup sugar
2 egg whites, at room temperature
¼ teaspoon cream of tartar

Soften gelatin in cold water for 5 minutes. Meanwhile, crush and strain fresh raspberries. Add boiling water to gelatin and stir until gelatin is completely dissolved. Add the crushed berries, lemon juice, and artificial sweetener and mix thoroughly. Chill mixture until it thickens and becomes syrupy, then beat at high speed with an electric mixer until foamy.

Beat the egg whites until foamy, add the cream of tartar, and continue beating until stiff but not dry. Very gently fold the raspberry mixture into the egg whites, being careful not to break down the whites. Turn the sponge pudding into a pretty serving dish and chill thoroughly.

20.1 grams of carbohydrate in entire recipe; if serving 6, each serving contains 3.4 grams of carbohydrate.

Chocolate Mousse

I've been told that my chocolate mousse with sugar is better than the one at Maxim's of Paris! This sugarless version is just as good.

Makes 8 servings

2 squares unsweetened chocolate
1 teaspoon unflavored gelatin
6 tablespoons cold water
4 extra-large eggs, at room temperature, separated
4 tablespoons chocolate extract
½ teaspoon mocha extract
Granulated artificial sweetener equal to 1¼ cups sugar
2 tablespoons dark rum
½ teaspoon cream of tartar

Melt chocolate over gentle heat or in a double boiler. Soften gelatin in cold water for 5 minutes. Add gelatin and water to melted chocolate. Separate the eggs, reserving the whites, and adding the yolks to the chocolate mixture. Heat the gelatin-chocolate mixture gently (avoid boiling). Remove from heat and add chocolate and mocha extracts, artificial sweetener, and rum. Mix thoroughly and chill till slightly thickened but not set.

Beat egg whites until foamy, add cream of tartar, and continue beating until stiff but not dry. Gently fold beaten egg whites into chilled chocolate mixture. Place in a decorative serving dish and refrigerate until thoroughly chilled.

17.4 grams of carbohydrate in entire recipe; if serving 8, each serving contains 2.2 grams of carbohydrate.

Lemon Mousse

Makes 2 servings

2 egg yolks, at room temperature
2½ tablespoons fresh lemon juice
1 teaspoon fresh lemon peel
Granulated artificial sweetener equal to ¼ cup sugar
¼ cup fat-free half-and-half
1 egg white, at room temperature
⅛ teaspoon cream of tartar
½ cup fresh strawberries, sliced
2 large, fresh, beautiful strawberries for garnish
Sprigs of fresh mint (optional)

Beat egg yolks at highest speed with an electric mixer until they are thick and lemon-colored. Beat in lemon juice and lemon peel. Do not use bottled lemon juice for this as the results will not be the same. Heat mixture over gentle heat or in the top of a double boiler until thick, stirring constantly. Let mixture cool and add artificial sweetener and half-and-half and mix in thoroughly.

Beat egg whites till foamy, add cream of tartar, and continue beating until stiff but not dry. Gently fold egg whites into lemon mixture. Fold in sliced strawberries.

Spoon mixture into 2 parfait or wineglasses. Top each with a fresh, whole strawberry and a sprig of fresh mint. Refrigerate the mousse and chill thoroughly.

14.5 grams of carbohydrate in entire recipe; if serving 2, each serving contains 7.3 grams of carbohydrate.

Tiramisu

I love fancy desserts. Don't you?

Makes 6 servings

½ recipe Butter Sponge Cake, baked in a 9-inch square pan (see page 43)
½ cup cooled strong espresso
6 teaspoons dark rum—4 teaspoons to mix with the coffee and 2 for the cream
3 extra-large eggs, at room temperature, separated
Granulated artificial sweetener equal to ½ cup and 2 tablespoons sugar
⅜ teaspoon cream of tartar
6 ounces ricotta, part-skim variety
2 ounces Neufchâtel cheese
2 tablespoons unsweetened cocoa powder

Bake the Butter Sponge Cake in advance. You can even freeze it for a few days. Cut the cake into strips the size of ladyfingers. Prepare the espresso, cool it, and mix in 4 teaspoons of the rum. With a pastry brush, brush the cake with the coffee-rum mixture and use the cake to line the bottom and sides of a 1½- to 2-quart bowl or rectangular dish.

Combine ¼ cup of the sweetener with the egg yolks and whisk over a very low flame in a heavy pot or alternately over a Flame Tamer until thickened and lemon-colored. Beat the egg whites until frothy, add the cream of tartar, and continue beating until stiff but not dry. Combine and beat together the ricotta, the Neufchâtel, sweetener equal to ¼ cup sugar, and 2 more teaspoons rum. Beat in the egg-yolk mixture, then very gently fold in the beaten egg whites. Spoon half of the cheese mixture over the prepared cake fingers.

Mix together 2 tablespoons of cocoa and sweetener equal to 2 tablespoons of sugar. Sift half of the cocoa mixture over the ricotta cream, then layer more of the coffee-brushed cake over the cream. Add the remainder of the cream over the cake. Sift the remaining cocoa mixture on the top. Refrigerate this for 6 to 8 hours before serving.

If you like dark chocolate, you will probably like the recipe this way. If you prefer milk chocolate, which is usually sweeter, you may want to mix one or two more tablespoons of sweetener with the cocoa. The people who tasted this seemed to break down into two distinct groups. Anyone who preferred dark chocolate said that the recipe was perfect the way it was. The milk chocolate lovers wanted the extra sweetener.

22.0 grams of carbohydrate in entire recipe; makes 6 servings, each serving contains 3.7 grams of carbohydrate.

Berry Misu

I personally like this better than tiramisu, which I really like. But the cream with the berries is wonderful.

Makes 6 servings

½ recipe Almond Sponge Cake (see page 45), baked in a 9-inch square pan
3 cups assorted berries, according to availability
2 teaspoons freshly grated lemon zest
Granulated artificial sweetener equal to approximately 1 cup sugar
3 extra-large eggs, at room temperature, separated
⅜ teaspoons cream of tartar
6 ounces ricotta, part-skim variety
2 ounces Neufchâtel cheese
4 teaspoons light rum
¼ teaspoon vanilla extract
1 perfect strawberry as a garnish

Bake the Almond Sponge Cake in advance. You can even freeze it for a few days. Cut the cake into strips the size of ladyfingers. Combine 3 cups of assorted berries. This can be any mixture of berries that is available in your market. Ideally, it would be lovely to have blueberries, strawberries, raspberries, and blackberries, but availability and price play a large factor. If all you can find is strawberries, then use only strawberries.

Mix the fruit with the lemon zest and the granulated artificial sweetener equal to approximately 6 to 8 tablespoons of sugar. This is a variable; taste the berries! Bear in mind that the cake is sweet, as is the ricotta cream. Combine ¼ cup of the sweetener with the egg yolks and whisk over a very low flame in a heavy pot or alternately over a Flame Tamer until thickened and lemon-colored. Whisk in 2 teaspoons light rum. Beat the egg whites until frothy, add the cream of tartar, and continue beating, until stiff but not dry. Combine and beat together the ricotta, the Neufchâtel, sweetener equal to ¼ cup of sugar, 2 more teaspoons of light rum, and ¼ teaspoon vanilla extract. Beat in the egg-yolk mixture, then very gently fold in the beaten egg whites.

Line the bottom and sides of a 1½- to 2-quart bowl or rectangular dish with the cake. The advantage of the rectangular dish is that it is easier to cut slices of the dessert. Put a layer of the berries in the dish followed by a layer of the ricotta cream. Add another layer of the cake followed by another layer of ricotta cream. Put a perfect strawberry on top for decoration, and refrigerate the Berry Misu for at least 6 hours before serving. This gives time for the flavors to blend.

64.0 grams of carbohydrate in entire recipe, makes 6 servings, each serving containing 10.7 grams of carbohydrate.

Ice Creams

Vanilla Ice Cream

Makes 8 servings

½ cup heavy cream
4 teaspoons unflavored gelatin
Dash of salt
2 extra-large eggs, at room temperature, separated
12 ounces ricotta cheese
1 tablespoon vanilla extract
Granulated artificial sweetener equal to ¾ cup sugar
¼ teaspoon cream of tartar

Combine cream, gelatin, salt, and egg yolks in the top of a double boiler or in a saucepan over gentle heat. Heat, stirring constantly, until gelatin dissolves and mixture is smooth, then place in a blender or food processor and add ricotta cheese, vanilla, and sweetener. Blend at high speed until smooth but not watery.

Beat egg whites until frothy, add cream of tartar, and beat until stiff but not dry. Empty ricotta mixture into egg whites and gently fold together. Rinse 2 ice trays with icy cold water, shake off excess, and fill with ice cream. Cover trays with aluminum foil and place in refrigerator freezing compartment at coldest setting for 1 hour. Lower temperature setting to normal after 1 hour and freeze until firm.

20.2 grams of carbohydrate in entire recipe; makes 2 trays of ice cream, each tray containing 10.1 grams of carbohydrate. If serving 8 (4 servings per tray), each serving contains 2.5 grams of carbohydrate.

Chocolate Ice Cream

Makes 8 servings

½ cup heavy cream
4 teaspoons unflavored gelatin
Dash of salt
2 extra-large eggs, at room temperature, separated
1 square unsweetened chocolate, melted
2 tablespoons plus 2 teaspoons chocolate extract
½ teaspoon vanilla extract
¼ teaspoon mocha extract
Granulated artificial sweetener equal to 1½ cups sugar
12 ounces ricotta cheese
Food coloring to make a chocolate-brown shade
¼ teaspoon cream of tartar

Follow method for Vanilla Ice Cream, adding chocolate and extracts to gelatin mixture after it has been removed from the heat, but before combining in the blender with the ricotta cheese. After the ricotta has been blended into the mixture, add food coloring as desired to deepen the chocolate color.

27.8 grams of carbohydrate in entire recipe; makes 2 trays of ice cream, each tray containing 13.9 grams of carbohydrate. If serving 8 (4 servings per tray), each serving contains 3.5 grams of carbohydrate.

Coffee Ice Cream

Makes 8 servings

½ cup heavy cream
4 teaspoons unflavored gelatin
Dash of salt
2 extra-large eggs, at room temperature, separated
1 tablespoon instant coffee
12 ounces ricotta cheese
Granulated artificial sweetener equal to ¼ cups sugar
¼ teaspoon cream of tartar

Follow instructions for Vanilla Ice Cream (page 85), adding the instant coffee to the blender before adding the ricotta.

20.1 grams of carbohydrate in entire recipe; makes 2 trays of ice cream, each tray containing 10.1 grams of carbohydrate. If serving 8 (4 servings per tray), each serving contains 2.5 grams of carbohydrate.

Maple Walnut Ice Cream

Makes 8 servings

½ cup heavy cream
4 teaspoons unflavored gelatin
Dash of salt
2 extra-large eggs, at room temperature, separated
12 ounces ricotta cheese
1½ teaspoons maple extract
20 drops vanilla extract

88 THE LOW-CARB GOURMET

Granulated artificial sweetener equal to ¾ cup sugar
¼ teaspoon cream of tartar
2 ounces finely chopped walnuts

Follow method for Vanilla Ice Cream (page 85), adding maple extract at the same time as vanilla. Fold in walnuts after you fold in egg white.

28.5 grams of carbohydrate in entire recipe; makes 2 trays of ice cream, each tray containing 14.3 grams of carbohydrate. If serving 8 (4 servings per tray), each serving contains 3.6 grams of carbohydrate.

Strawberry Ice Cream

Makes 8 servings

½ cup heavy cream
4 teaspoons unflavored gelatin
Dash of salt
2 extra-large eggs, at room temperature, separated
1½ teaspoons vanilla extract
Granulated artificial sweetener equal to 1 cup sugar
12 ounces ricotta cheese
1 cup sliced fresh strawberries
12 drops red food coloring
¼ teaspoon cream of tartar

Follow method for Vanilla Ice Cream (page 85), adding strawberries and food coloring to the blender *after* adding the ricotta.

32.2 grams of carbohydrate in entire recipe; makes 2 trays of ice cream, each tray containing 16.1 grams of carbohydrate. If serving 8 (4 servings per tray), each serving contains 4.0 grams of carbohydrate.

Granites

Coffee Granite

If you like espresso, try this delightful frozen variety.

Makes 6 servings

2 cups strong coffee, prepared from an Italian-roast blend
Granulated artificial sweetener equal to ½ cup sugar
1 cup cold water

Combine the coffee and the sweetener, stirring thoroughly to dissolve the sweetener. Mix in the remaining cup of cold water, and chill the coffee until cold.

Rinse 2 ice trays with icy cold water, shake off the excess, and fill with the cooled coffee.

Place the trays in your freezer and set a timer for 30 minutes.

When your timer rings, stir the granite to break up the ice crystals that will have formed around the edge of the tray. Return to the freezer, continuing to break up the ice crystals every thirty minutes for the first 2 hours, then every 15 minutes until the entire dessert has become coarsely crushed ice.

This dessert can be made a few hours in advance, but should not be made the night before or if you are not going to be at home, as you must continue to stir the ice every 15 minutes after it is ready to keep it from becoming solid. If you have an ice crusher, you can freeze this solid and then crush the flavored ice.

Serve the Coffee Granite from a crystal bowl or in individual wineglasses or parfait glasses.

Carbohydrate values for the Coffee Granite are so low they need not be counted at all.

Chocolate Granite

I know that nothing will please a chocolate lover except more chocolate.

Makes 6 servings

6 tablespoons imported Dutch cocoa, such as Droste
Granulated artificial sweetener equal to 6–8 tablespoons sugar
½ cup cold water
2½ cups boiling water
1 square (1 ounce) unsweetened chocolate, grated

Stir together the cocoa, sweetener, and cold water to make a paste. Add the boiling water and mix thoroughly until the sweetener and the cocoa are completely dissolved.

Cool the mixture and then follow remaining preparation instructions for Coffee Granite.

When the granite is half frozen, mix in the grated chocolate and continue freezing.

25.1 grams of carbohydrate in entire recipe; makes 2 trays of ice, each tray containing 12.6 grams of carbohydrate. If serving 6 (3 servings per tray), each serving contains 4.1 grams of carbohydrate.

Strawberry Granite

Pink and pretty.

Makes 6 servings

2 cups fresh, ripe strawberries, puréed in a blender
Granulated artificial sweetener equal to ½ cup sugar
1½ cups cold water
2 tablespoons freshly squeezed lemon juice

Combine all ingredients, then follow preparation for Coffee Granite (page 89).

26.6 grams of carbohydrate in entire recipe; makes 2 trays of ice, each tray containing 13.3 grams of carbohydrate. If serving 6, (3 servings per tray), each serving contains 4.4 grams of carbohydrate.

Zabaglione

Makes 4 servings

6 egg yolks
¼ cup dry sherry
¼ cup Chablis or similar dry white wine
Granulated artificial sweetener equal to 5–6 tablespoons sugar

Combine egg yolks and wines in the top of a double boiler. Keep heat very low so water in the lower boiler simmers, but does not boil. Beat the mixture very gently with a wire whisk, and keep moving the cooked zabaglione to the center of the pan and moving the uncooked part to the sides. Mixture will rise and thicken, but must not boil. Once the zabaglione has risen, remove from heat, and beat in artificial sweetener very briefly.

Serve immediately, while warm, in long-stemmed glasses.

2.7 grams of carbohydrate in entire recipe; if serving 4, each serving contains 0.7 grams of carbohydrate.

Frio, Frio

A quick, easy cooler.

Can be made to serve any number of people

Crushed ice
No-Cal Syrup—any flavor, or any other sugarless,
 no-carbohydrate syrup

Crush ice. This is easy to do in a blender if you first put in 1 full cup of water. Drain off excess water. Place crushed ice in a dessert dish. Pour any flavor syrup over the crushed ice and eat immediately with a spoon.

Carbohydrate values are so low they need not be counted at all.

NOTE: This is an inexpensive cooler. Frio is Spanish for cold. In Spanish-speaking countries and Spanish-speaking neighborhoods in New York, it is made with a paper cup full of crushed ice and sold on the streets. Another name for these is Sno-Cones or Snowballs. Fruit-flavored syrups are customarily used.

Ice Pops

Do you miss the ice pops you used to buy from the Good Humor man?

Makes 1 ice cube tray of ice pops

2 cups fruit-flavored dietetic soda
1 envelope artificially sweetened dietetic gelatin, same flavor as soda
Artificial sweetener equal to 1 cup sugar

Bring 1 cup of soda to a boil. Remove from heat and stir in gelatin. Mix until gelatin is dissolved, then add remaining soda and artificial sweetener. Chill gelatin mixture until cooled but not set. Pour into an ice cube tray—the plastic kind with individual cubes is good. Place a plastic toothpick in each section and freeze until solid.

To unmold, twist tray and ice pops should pop out. If necessary, place tray, bottom side up, under warm water for a moment. Store ice pops in a plastic bag in the freezer.

Negligible grams of carbohydrate in the entire recipe.

Some Sweet Diet Drinks

Vanilla Milk Shake

Do you still think that a cheeseburger and a milk shake make the best lunch of all?

Makes 3½ cups

¼ cup fat-free half-and-half
¼ cup cold water
12 ounces ricotta cheese, part-skim variety
4 ice cubes
2 generous teaspoons vanilla extract
Artificial sweetener equal to ¼ cup sugar

Place all ingredients in a blender and blend at highest speed until thoroughly mixed and frothy. Store in the refrigerator and use as desired from the blender container, blending it again 1 or 2 seconds before each use. This is an excellent way to get nourishment at times when you may not feel like eating, or at times when you are in a hurry, since it can be made the night before.

21.8 grams of carbohydrate in entire recipe; makes 3½ cups of milk shake when blended, each cup containing 6.2 grams of carbohydrate.

Vanilla Milk Shake—A More Dietetic Variation

This milk shake has even fewer carbohydrates and fewer calories. I personally prefer it.

Makes 3 cups

¼ cup fat-free half-and-half
½ cup cold water
6 ounces ricotta cheese, part-skim variety
4 ice cubes
1 teaspoon vanilla extract
Artificial sweetener equal to ¼ cup sugar

Follow directions for Vanilla Milk Shake.

14.0 grams of carbohydrate in entire recipe; makes 3 cups of milk shake when blended, each cup containing 4.7 grams of carbohydrate.

Coffee Milk Shake

A milk shake for the coffee lovers. Makes a quick, delicious breakfast.

Makes 3 cups

¼ cup fat-free half-and-half
½ cup cold water
6 ounces ricotta cheese, part-skim variety
4 ice cubes

1½ teaspoons instant coffee
Granulated artificial sweetener equal to 6 tablespoons sugar

Follow the directions for Vanilla Milk Shake (page 93), adding instant coffee to the blender with the other ingredients.

14.5 grams of carbohydrate in entire recipe; makes 3 cups of milk shake when blended, each cup containing 4.8 grams of carbohydrate.

Banana Milk Shake

Makes 3 cups

¼ cup fat-free half-and-half
½ cup cold water
6 ounces ricotta cheese, part-skim variety
4 ice cubes
1 tablespoon banana extract
¼ teaspoon vanilla extract
¼ teaspoon lemon juice
Granulated artificial sweetener equal to 6 tablespoons sugar

Follow directions for Vanilla Milk Shake (page 93), adding the banana extract to the blender with the other ingredients.

13.9 grams of carbohydrate in entire recipe; makes 3 cups when blended, each cup containing 4.6 grams of carbohydrate.

Chocolate Egg Cream

Makes 1 serving

Ice cubes
1 cup sugarless chocolate soda, chilled
2 teaspoons fat-free half-and-half

96 THE LOW-CARB GOURMET

Fill a tall glass with ice cubes. Pour the soda over the ice cubes. Mix in the cream and serve immediately with a straw.

0.5 grams of carbohydrate in entire recipe; makes 1 serving.

Natalie's Iced Coffee

My friend Natalie has this coffee for breakfast every morning.

Makes 4 servings

Ice cubes
3 cups strong coffee, regular or decaffeinated
4 teaspoons fat-free half-and-half
2 teaspoons vanilla extract
Artificial sweetener to taste

Fill 4 tall glasses with ice cubes. Mix together the coffee, half-and-half, and vanilla and fill the 4 glasses. Serve artificial sweetener alongside the iced coffee and let each person sweeten the coffee to taste.

3.2 grams of carbohydrate in entire recipe; if serving 4, each serving contains 0.8 grams of carbohydrate.

Frozen Mochachino

Did you ever realize what a sugar fix you are getting when you order a Frozen Mochachino in a coffeehouse or restaurant?

Makes 3 cups

2 cups double-strength chilled chocolate hazelnut coffee*
1 tablespoon and 1 teaspoon unsweetened cocoa
3 tablespoons fat-free half-and-half
Artificial sweetener equal to ½ cup sugar
1 full tray of ice cubes

Put all of the ingredients in a blender that is capable of crushing ice or alternately in a smoothie maker and blend thoroughly until the ice cubes are crushed and your ingredients are well combined. Depending on your taste, you can add a little more fat-free half-and-half or extra sweetener. I like very strong coffee or tea, but it may be too strong for you; this is an easy recipe to adjust to your own taste. Serve in tall stemmed glasses.

8.5 grams of carbohydrate in entire recipe; makes 3 cups, each cup containing 2.8 grams of carbohydrate.

NOTE: If you have the time or plan ahead, you can make regular-strength coffee and freeze one tray of coffee cubes and chill the rest of the coffee, then proceed to follow the recipe. I like it even better with the coffee cubes.

---

*This would also work well with chocolate almond coffee, but if neither chocolate hazelnut coffee nor chocolate almond coffee are available in your area, you can make double-strength coffee with any good-quality coffee. Just add more unsweetened cocoa powder, but remember to add 3 grams of carbohydrate for each tablespoon of cocoa used. This is so low-carbohydrate anyway, when compared to the sugared variety, that you probably can still have it, and on a hot summer's day it's delightful.

III.

To Begin a Meal: Hors D'Oeuvres, Appetizers, and Soups

Liver Pâté   101
Melon with Prosciutto   102
Rumaki   103
Roquefort Grapes   104
Stuffed Mushrooms   105
Shrimp Cocktails   106
Hot Shrimp Cocktails   107
Consommé with Sherry   108
Stracciatella Soup   108
Gazpacho Soup   109
Easy Borscht   110
Fresh Mushroom Soup—Hot or Cold   111
French Onion Soup   112
Bisque of Zucchini   112
Frothy Greek Lemon Soup   113
Cold Lemon-Sorrel Soup   114
Chilled Melon Soup   115
Cold Fresh Raspberry Soup   116
Strawberry Soup   116

To Begin a Meal: Hors d'Oeuvres, Appetizers, and Soups

The appetizers included here can be used either to begin a meal or as hors d'oeuvres for parties. I have also included several of my favorite soup recipes, and if you have never tasted cold soup, you are in for a treat. Watch for other recipes elsewhere in this book such as scampi, grilled tomatoes with cheese, and various stuffed vegetables, which can also be used as a first course.

Liver Pâté

Makes 5 servings

1 pound chicken livers
2 tablespoons whipped butter
4 tablespoons extra-virgin olive oil
1 large onion, finely chopped
2 tablespoons dry sherry
1 tablespoon Calvados, applejack, or Cognac
1 tablespoon fat-free half-and-half
1 teaspoon salt (or to taste)
1/4 teaspoon freshly ground black pepper
1/2 teaspoon Madras curry powder (page 20)
Lettuce leaves or apple slices for garnish

Wash and dry the livers, cut in halves, and set aside. Melt 1 tablespoon of the butter and 2 tablespoons of oil in a large nonstick skillet. Add the onions and sauté over medium heat 10 to 12 minutes, or until soft and slightly golden. Transfer onions and pan juices to a blender or food processor. In the same skillet, melt remaining butter and oil over high heat, add the livers, and cook 4 to 5 minutes, turning frequently. The livers should be thoroughly browned outside and cooked inside (slice one to check). Add the livers and pan juices to the onions in the blender, then put in sherry, Calvados, half-and-half, salt, pepper, and curry powder. Blend at high speed until pâté is completely smooth. A rubber spatula is helpful for this job. Place pâté in a crock and cover with plastic wrap to keep if from darkening. Refrigerate for at least 3 to 4 hours. Serve on lettuce leaves or thin slices of apple.

25.5 grams of carbohydrate in entire recipe; if serving 5, each serving contains 5.1 grams of carbohydrate.

Melon with Prosciutto

A perennial favorite.

Makes 4 servings

1 whole cantaloupe, about 5 inches in diameter
¼ pound Italian prosciutto, preferably imported (page 22)
Freshly ground black pepper
Lemon or lime wedges, if desired

Slice the cantaloupe into 8 wedges. Wrap a slice of the prosciutto around each piece. Place 2 wedges of the cantaloupe on each of four plates and serve with a pepper mill so that people can grind some fresh black pepper over their own servings. Lemon or lime wedges may be added to each plate, if desired.

28.0 grams of carbohydrate in entire recipe; if serving 4, each serving contains 7.0 grams of carbohydrate.

NOTE: If cantaloupe is out of season, you may substitute any melon that is available.

Rumaki

Polynesian rumaki can be used as an appetizer to start a meal or as an hors d'oeuvre for a party.

Makes 18 skewers

½ pound bacon
½ pound chicken livers
2 tablespoons soy sauce
2 tablespoons dry sherry
1 tablespoon peanut oil
1 clove garlic, minced
Slice of fresh gingerroot, minced
Artificial sweetener equal to 2 teaspoons sugar
9 water chestnuts, fresh or canned

Partially fry or broil the bacon, cut each piece in half, and set aside. Cut each chicken liver in half and remove any bits of tendon. Combine the soy sauce, sherry, oil, garlic, ginger, and artificial sweetener. Place the precooked bacon and the livers in the soy-sherry marinade for at least 30 minutes, or 1 hour if time is available. Slice each water chestnut in half. Wrap a piece of marinated chicken liver around a slice of water chestnut, then wrap a piece of bacon around the liver, and spear with a dampened toothpick or tiny skewer. Repeat until all pieces are wrapped and speared. Broil the rumaki about 4 inches from the source of heat for 4 to 5 minutes, turning several times. The liver should remain pink inside. Serve hot.

25.3 grams of carbohydrate in entire recipe; makes 18 rumaki, each one containing 1.4 grams of carbohydrate.

Roquefort Grapes

The idea for these came from Martha Stewart, who has taught all of us so much. I've reduced the saturated fats and they still taste delicious.

Makes 50 grapes

1 10-ounce package of almonds, pecans, or walnuts
1 8-ounce package of Neufchâtel cheese
2 ounces French Roquefort cheese
2 tablespoons fat-free half-and-half
1 pound seedless grapes, red and/or green, washed and dried

Preheat oven to 275° F. Line a baking sheet with aluminum foil. Spread the nuts on sheet and bake. If using almonds, they should be a light golden brown color while walnuts or pecans should smell toasted but not burnt. Chop the nuts coarsely in a food processor or with a nut chopper. Put them on a plate or, if the baking sheet has cooled, you can use that. In a bowl, combine the Neufchâtel cheese, the Roquefort cheese, and the half-and-half. Beat with an electric mixer until smooth. Drop the dried grapes into the cheese mixture to coat them. When coated, roll them in the toasted nuts until they are coated. Cover a tray with waxed paper and place the grapes on this tray. Refrigerate until serving time. (No, you may not pop more than one of these in your mouth while preparing them! I know it's tempting.)

121.2 grams of carbohydrate in entire recipe if using almonds; makes 50 grapes, each containing 2.4 grams of carbohydrate.
101.2 grams of carbohydrate in entire recipe if using

pecans or walnuts; makes 50 grapes, each containing 2.0 grams of carbohydrate.

Stuffed Mushrooms

These are just another excuse to use my favorite sauce. I admit to loving portobello mushrooms also; wait until you taste the combination. Two of these would be a lovely light luncheon dish when served with a salad. (Carry a breath spray along in your pocket.)

Makes 4 mushrooms

4 medium-size portobello mushrooms
2 tablespoons extra-virgin olive oil
2 teaspoons balsamic vinegar
½ cup ricotta cheese, part-skim variety
2 tablespoons Pesto Sauce (see page 262)
2 tablespoons grated Parmesan cheese

Preheat oven to 425° F. Remove the stems from the mushrooms and set them aside for another use. We are using only the mushroom caps. Wipe the mushroom caps with a damp paper towel; do not put them under the faucet to wash them! They are like a sponge and will absorb too much water. Whisk together the oil and vinegar and lightly brush the mushroom caps on both sides with this mixture. Mix together the ricotta with the Pesto Sauce and divide the mixture among the 4 mushroom caps. Sprinkle the tops of each mushroom with ½ tablespoon grated Parmesan cheese. These should be placed in a nonstick pan or on nonstick aluminum foil and baked in the oven for approximately 18 minutes. Remove from the oven and enjoy them.

16.4 grams of carbohydrate in entire recipe; makes 4 mushrooms, each mushroom containing 4.1 grams of carbohydrate.

Shrimp Cocktails

Makes 6 servings

1½ pounds large raw shrimp, cleaned and deveined
1 cup water
½ cup dry white wine
1 small bay leaf
¼ teaspoon thyme
¾ teaspoon salt
4 peppercorns
6 medium-sized shells
Lettuce leaves
Any shrimp sauce recipe (see Chapter Ten)
Wedge of lemon

Place the shrimp in a saucepan with the water, wine, bay leaf, thyme, salt, and peppercorns. It's nice to tie the spices in a little cheesecloth and then add them to the pot. Cover the pan, bring to a boil, then lower the flame, and simmer for about 8 minutes. Do not overcook the shrimp. Remove shrimp from the liquid, drain thoroughly, and chill.

To serve, divide the shrimp among 6 seashells, each lined with a lettuce leaf. Spoon some of the sauce over each portion or serve sauce separately in another dish for dipping. Garnish with a wedge of lemon.

7.1 grams of carbohydrate in entire recipe; if serving 6, each serving contains 1.2 grams of carbohydrate plus the grams for your chosen sauce.

Hot Shrimp Cocktails

Try a change from the usual cold shrimp cocktail.

Makes 6 servings

1½ pounds raw shrimp, cleaned and deveined
1 cup water
½ cup dry white wine
1 small bay leaf
¼ teaspoon thyme
¾ teaspoon salt
4 peppercorns
1 large or 2 small cloves garlic, minced
2 tablespoons butter, melted, and 4 tablespoons extra-virgin olive oil
¼ cup imported Parmesan cheese
Salt and freshly ground pepper to taste
6 medium-sized shells or ramekins
Minced parsley

Place shrimp in a saucepan with water, wine, bay leaf, thyme, salt, and peppercorns. Cover pan, bring to a boil, and simmer for 6 to 7 minutes. Remove shrimp from the liquid and drain thoroughly. Preheat oven to 425° F. Distribute shrimp evenly among 6 shells or ramekins, then add the minced garlic to the melted butter and oil, and spoon a tablespoonful over each serving. Sprinkle with Parmesan cheese, salt, and freshly ground pepper to taste, and bake about 5 minutes. The butter and oil should be sizzling. Sprinkle with minced parsley and serve immediately.

9.0 grains of carbohydrate in entire recipe; if serving 6, each serving contains 1.5 grams of carbohydrate.

108   THE LOW-CARB GOURMET

Consommé with Sherry

Precede a heavy dinner with a light, delicately flavored broth.

Serves 4

4 cups beef broth, fresh, canned, or made from a cube or powder
4–8 teaspoons dry sherry

Prepare beef broth as directed from the can or package mix you are using. Pour steaming hot broth into soup cups. To each cup add 1 or 2 teaspoons dry sherry and stir. Serve very hot.

2.2 grams of carbohydrate in entire recipe; if serving 4, each serving contains 0.6 grams of carbohydrate.

Stracciatella Soup

A popular Italian soup.

Serves 5

2 eggs
4 tablespoons freshly grated Parmesan cheese
4 cups chicken broth, fresh, canned, or made from a cube or powder
4 tablespoons freshly minced parsley
Salt and freshly ground pepper to taste

Beat eggs thoroughly. Add cheese and a few tablespoons of unheated broth and beat together with the eggs. Heat remaining broth to boiling point, and add the egg-cheese mixture slowly, stirring constantly. Simmer the soup for about 5 minutes, stirring constantly. Remove from flame, stir in minced parsley, and ladle soup into hot bowls or soup cups. Additional cheese may be added, if desired.

3.4 grams of carbohydrate in entire recipe; if serving 5, each serving contains 0.7 grams of carbohydrate.

Gazpacho Soup

This is really a soup salad.

Serves 6

3 very ripe tomatoes, peeled, seeded, and sliced
1 green pepper, seeded and sliced
1 medium cucumber, peeled, seeded, and sliced
½ onion, sliced
½ cup chilled beef broth
3 tablespoons wine vinegar
2 tablespoons olive oil
1 large clove garlic, minced
½ teaspoon basil
Salt and freshly ground pepper to taste—depends on degree of salt in broth
⅛ teaspoon ground celery seed
⅛–¼ teaspoon ground cumin

Place all ingredients in a blender or food processor and blend at moderate speed until vegetables are just chopped. Do not overblend. Chill thoroughly until time to serve. Serve in chilled cups or bowls. Add 1 or 2 ice cubes to each bowl, if desired.

43.2 grams of carbohydrate in entire recipe; if serving 6, each serving contains 7.2 grams of carbohydrate.

Easy Borscht

Making borscht with canned beets is much easier than using fresh beets and tastes just as good.

Makes 12 servings

One 1-pound can whole beets
2 quarts cold water
¼ teaspoon salt or more to taste
Artificial sweetener equal to 5 tablespoons sugar
4 eggs
Sour cream, 50 percent reduced fat

Grate the canned beets, reserving the liquid from the can. Bring the water to a boil, add beets, beet liquid, and salt. Return to boil, then lower flame, and simmer 5 minutes. Remove from heat and stir in artificial sweetener. Beat the eggs thoroughly with a wire whisk. Add 1 cup of the hot liquid to eggs, whisking thoroughly as you pour, then whisk egg mixture thoroughly into the hot soup. Chill soup thoroughly. Serve with sour cream on the side and let people help themselves or add a dollop on top of each serving.

62.5 grams of carbohydrate in entire recipe; if serving 12, each serving contains 5.2 grams of carbohydrate. Add 1.5 grams of carbohydrate for each tablespoon of sour cream.

Fresh Mushroom Soup—Hot or Cold

Makes 6 servings

1 pound fresh white mushrooms
2¼ cups double-strength chicken broth
½ cup fat-free half-and-half
¼ cup dry sherry
Salt and freshly ground pepper to taste
Ground nutmeg
Minced parsley

Wipe the mushrooms with a damp paper towel and coarsely slice them. Place them in a blender container, add 1 cup of the chicken broth, and purée the mixture. Pour it into the top of a double boiler or into a saucepan placed over a gentle heat. Add the remaining 1¼ cups of chicken broth, the half-and-half, and the dry sherry. Season with salt, pepper, and nutmeg to taste. Bring the soup to a boil over low heat, then cover it with plastic wrap or aluminum foil to prevent a skin from forming over it.

This soup can be made in advance and reheated, but do not cook it further. Since this is a rich soup, it is best served in soup cups. Sprinkle the top with the minced parsley. This soup may also be chilled in the refrigerator and served cold. It's even better than vichyssoise.

37.7 grams of carbohydrate in entire recipe; if serving 6, each serving contains 6.3 grams of carbohydrate.

French Onion Soup

Did you ever eat onion soup at Les Halles in Paris at four A.M.? I was twenty-one when I took my first trip to Europe, supposedly to go to the Sorbonne, but I never even registered for the course. My happiest memory is eating a soup very much like this one.

Makes 8 servings

6 small onions
2 tablespoons extra-virgin olive oil and 1 tablespoon whipped butter
1 teaspoon flour
6 cups beef broth
½ cup very dry white wine or vermouth
1 tablespoon Cognac (optional)
Salt and freshly ground pepper to taste
3 tablespoons grated Swiss Gruyère cheese
Additional grated Parmesan cheese

Slice the onions very thin. Sauté them in the butter and oil until lightly browned. Mix in the flour and cook for 2 or 3 minutes more. Stir in the beef broth, wine, and Cognac. Season to taste with salt and freshly ground black pepper. Gently simmer the soup for 15 to 20 minutes. Add the Swiss cheese and continue simmering until the cheese melts. Stir frequently while the cheese melts. When serving, sprinkle each serving with additional grated Parmesan cheese.

36.8 grams of carbohydrate in entire recipe; if serving 8, each serving contains 4.6 grams of carbohydrate. Add 0.2 grams of carbohydrate for each tablespoon of grated Parmesan used.

Bisque of Zucchini

Makes 4 servings

1 pound zucchini, unpeeled
1 small onion, coarsely chopped
1 stalk celery, coarsely chopped
5 sprigs parsley
3 cups chicken broth, fresh, canned, or made from a cube or powder
2 egg yolks
2 tablespoons fat-free half-and-half
2 tablespoons cold water
Salt and freshly ground pepper to taste

Wash zucchini thoroughly and chop coarsely without peeling. Place in a heavy saucepan with remaining vegetables and chicken broth. Bring the mixture to a boil and simmer uncovered for 40 minutes. Place the mixture in a blender or food processor and blend until smooth, then return it to the pot it was cooked in. Combine the egg yolks with the half-and-half and water and a few tablespoons of the hot soup, then stir this mixture thoroughly into the soup. Reheat the soup if necessary, but do not allow it to boil. Add salt and pepper to taste.

26.8 grams of carbohydrate in entire recipe; if serving 4, each serving contains 6.7 grams of carbohydrate.

Frothy Greek Lemon Soup

This light-as-air lemony soup is a delightful way to start a meal. Try it as a prelude to Shish Kebab.

Makes 6 servings

4 cups chicken broth, fresh, canned, or made from a cube or powder
4 extra-large eggs, at room temperature, separated
½ teaspoon cream of tartar
4 tablespoons lemon juice
6 thin slices of lemon

Bring the chicken broth to a boil. Meanwhile, beat the egg whites until foamy, add the cream of tartar, and continue beating until stiff but not dry. Beat the egg yolks with the lemon juice. Gently fold the egg whites into the yolks and gradually, with a wire whisk, stir in half of the boiling chicken broth. Immediately pour the mixture back into the remaining broth and continue heating over low heat, stirring constantly until thickened. Pour into soup cups and garnish with the thin slices of lemon.

10.8 grams of carbohydrate in entire recipe; if serving 6, each serving contains 1.8 grams of carbohydrate.

Cold Lemon-Sorrel Soup

This is a lemony version of the usual cold sorrel soup.

Makes 10 servings

1 pound sorrel leaves
2 teaspoons salt
2 quarts water
¼ cup fresh lemon juice
Artificial sweetener equal to ¼ cup sugar
3 eggs
Sour cream, 50 percent reduced fat

Trim the heavy stems from the sorrel, then wash and dry it. This is easily done by scrubbing your sink thoroughly and then filling it with cold water. Place the sorrel in the water and move it around with your hands. Change the water once or twice. Dry on paper towels or in a salad spinner. Shred the leaves and place in a heavy enamel saucepan with salt and water. Bring to a boil and cook for 20 minutes. Add lemon juice and cook 10 minutes more. Remove from heat and add artificial sweetener. Beat the eggs thoroughly with a wire whisk, then mix with 1 cup of the hot liquid, whisking thoroughly as you pour the liquid into the eggs. Whisk this egg mixture into the rest of the soup. Chill thoroughly. You can add sour cream to all of the soup beforehand, but I prefer to serve the sour cream on the side so people can help themselves or else to add a dollop on top of each serving.

24.1 grams of carbohydrate in entire recipe; if serving 10, each serving contains 2.4 grams of carbohydrate. Add 1.5 grams of carbohydrate for each tablespoon of sour cream.

Chilled Melon Soup

For an appetizer or for dessert.

Makes 4 servings

1½ pounds ripe cantaloupe, Spanish melon, or Casaba melon
2 tablespoons dry sherry
1½ teaspoons fresh lime juice
Artificial sweetener equal to 2 tablespoons sugar
Fresh mint to garnish

Remove all seeds from the melon and trim away rind. Cut melon into small chunks and place in a blender. Add sherry, lime juice, and sweetener and blend until smooth. Pour the mixture into a plastic container or glass jar, cover, and refrigerate until very cold. Mix the soup thoroughly before putting into serving cups as it separates upon standing. To serve, garnish each soup cup with a sprig of fresh mint and 1 or 2 melon balls.

26.6 grams of carbohydrate in entire recipe; if serving 4, each serving contains 6.7 grams of carbohydrate.

Cold Fresh Raspberry Soup

This sweet, delicious soup can be served as either an appetizer or as a dessert.

Makes 6 servings

2 cups fresh raspberries
2 cups cold water
½ cup red wine
½ cup sour cream, 50 percent reduced fat
Artificial sweetener equal to ½ cup sugar
Fresh mint to garnish

Crush and strain the fresh raspberries. Mix in the water, wine, sour cream, and artificial sweetener. A wire whisk is good for this job. Chill thoroughly until serving time. Serve icy cold in chilled soup cups and garnish with 2 or 3 fresh raspberries and a sprig of fresh mint.

46.6 grams of carbohydrate in entire recipe; if serving 6, each serving contains 7.8 grams of carbohydrate.

Strawberry Soup

Again, serve as an appetizer or for dessert.

Makes 6 servings

2 cups ripe strawberries
½ cup sour cream, 50 percent reduced fat
2 cups cold water
½ cup Bordeaux or similar red wine

Artificial sweetener equal to ½ cup sugar
Fresh mint to garnish

Wash and hull the strawberries, then place in a blender. Add sour cream and blend to a purée. Empty the mixture into a heavy saucepan and add water and wine. Heat the mixture very slowly over very low heat, stirring constantly with a wooden spoon. Do not let the soup boil. Remove from heat and stir in the artificial sweetener. Chill the soup, and when serving, garnish each plate with a few whole strawberries and a sprig of fresh mint.

35.8 grams of carbohydrate in entire recipe; if serving 6, each serving contains 6.0 grams of carbohydrate.

IV.

Meats: The Backbone of Low-Carbohydrate Diets

Beef Kebabs 122
Beef Stroganoff 123
Cheese-Filled Hamburgers 124
Herb-Crusted Boneless Beef Roast 124
Herb-Crusted Leg of Lamb 126
Italian Meat and Cheese Casserole 127
Meat-Crusted Pizza 128
London Broil with Boursin 130
Soy-Glazed London Broil 130
Roquefort-Topped Steak 132
Steak with Chicken-Liver Sauce 133
Steak with Mushroom Sauce 134
Veal Scallops with Chives and Cheese 135
Party Veal Scallops 136
Veal Chops in Mustard Sauce 137
Grilled Lamb Chops or
   Lamb Steaks with Mint Pesto 138
Lamb Shish Kebab 139
Sautéed Calf's Liver 140

Meats: The Backbone of Low-Carbohydrate Diets

Meats are the backbone of a low-carbohydrate diet because they contain *no* carbohydrates and are high in protein. At the same time, while steaks, roasts, hamburgers, and chops are delicious in themselves, one can become very bored eating them plain all the time. In this chapter, I have presented some low-carbohydrate variations on ways to prepare meats. Many of these recipes require very little more time and effort than just broiling a steak, yet they are interesting, tasty, and should keep anyone from becoming bored.

Beef Kebabs

Good for the barbecue, too.

Makes 2 servings

1 pound sirloin steak
1 cup dry red wine
1 onion, chopped
1 carrot, chopped
2 shallots, chopped
6 peppercorns
Coarse salt
Pinch of thyme
1 bay leaf
3 cloves
2 tablespoons Cognac
12 medium-size mushroom caps
6 tiny, white onions, parboiled for 10 minutes
1 tablespoon extra-virgin olive oil

Cut meat into 2-inch cubes and marinate in a mixture of the wine, onion, carrot, shallots, peppercorns, salt, thyme, bay leaf, cloves, and Cognac. Allow meat to marinate 48 hours, turning the cubes occasionally, then drain, and dry each piece carefully in paper towels. Thread meat on skewers, alternating with mushroom caps and parboiled onions. Using a pastry brush, brush skewers with oil.

Broil under a high flame, turning until meat is brown on all sides but still rare inside.

20.0 grams of carbohydrate in entire recipe; if serving 2, each serving contains 10.0 grams of carbohydrate.

Beef Stroganoff

Makes 4 servings

1½ pounds fillet of beef
3 tablespoons extra-virgin olive oil
2 teaspoons whipped butter
½ small onion, thinly sliced
4 medium-size fresh mushrooms, thinly sliced
⅓ cup dry white wine
1 cup sour cream, 50 percent reduced fat
Salt and freshly ground pepper to taste
Dash of garlic powder
Dash of dry mustard
1 tablespoon and 1 teaspoon lemon juice
Few dashes of Worcestershire sauce
Minced parsley

Cut meat into very thin slices, or have butcher do it. Heat 2 tablespoons of the oil along with butter in a large, heavy skillet. Get it as hot as possible, but do not let it burn. Sauté the beef slices in the hot fat very quickly—1 or 2 minutes per side. When delicately browned on both sides, remove to a hot platter. Add remaining oil to the skillet and sauté the onion slices until transparent. Add mushrooms, and sauté a few minutes longer. Add the wine and bring to a boil. Lower heat, add sour cream, salt, pepper, garlic powder, mustard, lemon juice, and Worcestershire sauce and stir well. Heat the sauce over a low flame, warming it thoroughly, but do not allow it to boil as this would curdle the sour cream. Return meat to pan and warm the entire dish for about another minute. Sprinkle with fresh parsley as a garnish when serving.

32.3 grams of carbohydrate in entire recipe; if serving 4, each serving contains 8.1 grams of carbohydrate.

NOTE: Try substituting turkey or chicken cut for scallopini for the beef, but do not pound it.

Cheese-Filled Hamburgers

The lowly hamburger becomes a sophisticate.

Makes 4 servings

2 pounds lean ground beef
Salt and freshly ground pepper to taste
Dash of garlic powder
4 tablespoons finely chopped onion
½ cup freshly chopped parsley
4 ounces French Roquefort cheese, crumbled
Strips of broiled bacon (optional)

Combine meat with salt, pepper, garlic powder, onion, and parsley. Shape meat into 4 elongated, flat hamburger patties, each about double the usual length. Sprinkle with crumbled Roquefort cheese. Fold each patty in half, shaping into 4 nice, fat hamburgers. Panbroil or broil to desired state of doneness. The cheese will melt throughout the meat and flavor it. Top with strips of broiled bacon, if desired.

6.0 grams of carbohydrate in entire recipe; if serving 4, each serving contains 1.5 grams of carbohydrate. Add 0.2 grams of carbohydrate for each thin slice of bacon.

Herb-Crusted Boneless Beef Roast

The herb crust really flavors the meat beautifully.

Makes 6 servings

Meats

3 pounds boneless beef roast, cut from the round or rib
3 tablespoons extra-virgin olive oil
3 large cloves fresh garlic
3 tablespoons fresh rosemary leaves
3 tablespoons fresh thyme leaves
¼ teaspoon herbs de Provence (page 16)
1 carrot, coarsely cut into chunks, to flavor the drippings
1 onion, coarsely cut into chunks, to flavor the drippings
Salt and freshly ground pepper to taste

Preheat oven to 425° F. In a food processor bowl, with the motor running, chop the garlic. Stop the motor and add the thyme and rosemary leaves and continue chopping. Mix in the oil and the herbs de Provence. This mixture can be chopped by hand if you have no food processor; it just will take a bit more time. Coat the beef with this mixture, coating all sides of the meat, and place on a rack in your roasting pan. Roast for 15 minutes at 425° F., then lower the oven temperature to 325° F. Strew the carrot and onion in the bottom of the pan to flavor the drippings, and continue roasting the meat at 325° F. until your meat thermometer registers 120° F.–125° F. for rare meat, 130° F.–135° F. for medium rare. This will take about 15 to 20 minutes per pound, but check your meat thermometer because this depends upon the shape of the meat.

Remove from the oven when the meat is cooked to your taste. Remember that the meat will continue to cook a little even while out of the oven. Allow the roast to rest for ten to fifteen minutes in a warm place. A favorite trick of mine to have hot rare roast beef for a second meal is to check the temperature closer to the ends if you know there is enough for two meals. Then slice the meat from each end the first night, leaving the center piece, which is the rarest part of the meat. The second night, put the meat back in the oven again at 325° F. until the center of the meat registers the way you enjoyed it the first night; that way you can have rare or medium-rare roast beef for a second night. Discard the carrot pieces and onion pieces from the drippings and place the drippings in a fat separator cup (a cup with an upper and lower spout). Enjoy a small amount of the lean, well-flavored drippings on your meat.

4.2 grams of carbohydrate in entire recipe; if serving 6, each serving contains 0.7 grams of carbohydrate.

Herb-Crusted Boneless Leg of Lamb

This is similar to Herb-Crusted Beef, but with a slight change in the herb mixture.

Makes 6 servings

3 pounds boneless leg of lamb
3 tablespoons extra-virgin olive oil
4 large cloves fresh garlic
3 tablespoons fresh rosemary leaves
3 tablespoons fresh thyme leaves
¼ cup fresh mint leaves
½ teaspoon Poissonnade (This is a French herb mixture for fish, which I feel balances out the stronger taste of lamb better than the other blend of herbs de Provence. If you're lucky enough to be able to obtain spring lamb, which has a more delicate flavor, you can cut the amount you're using down to ¼ teaspoon.)
1 carrot, coarsely cut into chunks, to flavor the drippings
1 onion, coarsely cut into chunks, to flavor the drippings
Salt and freshly ground pepper to taste

Preheat oven to 450° F. The method used here is similar to the method used to prepare the herb mixture for Herb-Crusted Beef. In a food processor bowl, with the motor running, chop the garlic. Stop the motor and add the rosemary leaves, thyme leaves, and mint leaves and continue chopping. Mix in the oil and the Poissonnade. This mixture can be chopped by hand if you have no food processor; it will just take a bit more time.

Coat the lamb with this mixture, coating all sides of the meat, and place on a rack in your roasting pan. Roast at 450° F. for 15 minutes to sear the meat, then lower the oven temperature to 350° F. Strew the carrot and onion in the bottom of the pan to flavor the drippings, and continue roasting at 350° F. until your meat thermometer registers 147° F.–150° F. for medium rare or 160° F.–165° F. for well done.

Remove from the oven when the meat is cooked to your taste. Remember that the meat will continue to cook a little even while out of the oven. Allow the meat to rest for 20 minutes in a warm place. Discard the carrot and onion pieces from the drippings and place the drippings in a fat separator cup (a cup with an upper and lower spout). Enjoy a small amount of the lean, well-flavored drippings on your meat. Season the lamb with salt and pepper to taste and serve it on warmed plates.

5.0 grams of carbohydrate in entire recipe; if serving 6, each serving contains 0.8 grams of carbohydrate.

Italian Meat and Cheese Casserole

A delicious meal in one dish.

Makes 4 servings

1 medium eggplant
3 tablespoons olive oil
2 teaspoons salt
½ teaspoon freshly ground black pepper
1 pound very lean ground beef
¼ pound chicken livers, diced
⅛ teaspoon garlic powder
¼ cup grated Parmesan cheese
6 ounces mozzarella cheese, thinly sliced, part-skim variety
1 tablespoon extra-virgin olive oil
1 tablespoon whipped butter

Preheat oven to 350° F. Peel eggplant and slice in thin slices. Place the oil in a heavy skillet and fry eggplant on both sides until golden brown. Sprinkle with 1 teaspoon of the salt and pepper. Sauté meat and diced chicken livers for 5 minutes, stirring constantly. Remove from heat and mix in garlic powder, 1 tablespoon of the Parmesan cheese, and remaining salt and pepper.

In a greased, pretty, 1-quart casserole, arrange a layer of eggplant, then a layer of meat, then a layer of mozzarella cheese. Repeat until all ingredients are used, ending with a layer of eggplant. Top with remaining Parmesan cheese and dot with butter and oil. Bake at 350° F. for 1 hour. Serve immediately from the casserole.

22.9 grams of carbohydrate in entire recipe; if serving 4, each serving contains 5.7 grams of carbohydrate.

Meat-Crusted Pizza

Who needs a fattening bread crust on pizza anyway?

Makes 6 servings

Crust

1 pound very lean ground beef
1 egg
½ small onion, finely chopped
1 small clove garlic, finely chopped
1 teaspoon salt
¼ teaspoon black pepper
2 tablespoons grated Parmesan cheese
¼ teaspoon fennel seed

Meats

Filling

¾ cup Italian plum tomatoes, drained and chopped
½ teaspoon crushed red pepper
¼ teaspoon oregano
¼ teaspoon basil
Salt and freshly ground pepper to taste

Topping

6 ounces mozzarella cheese, part-skim variety
2 hot Italian sausages
¼ teaspoon oregano
3 tablespoons grated Parmesan cheese

Mix together the beef, egg, onion, garlic, salt, black pepper, cheese, and fennel seed. Press the mixture into a 9-inch pie plate to form a shell. Preheat the oven to 375° F. Bake the pie shell 15 minutes, then pour off any fat that may have collected. If your meat was lean, you should have hardly any fat.

Mix together the tomatoes, red pepper, oregano, basil, and salt and pepper to taste. Spread the flavored tomatoes over the pie shell. Arrange the mozzarella in thin slices over the tomatoes. Cook the sausages 5 minutes, then drain, and slice into ½-inch rounds. Arrange sausage rounds over cheese. Sprinkle the pizza with another ¼ teaspoon of oregano, then with grated Parmesan cheese. You may add any other toppings you desire to this. Bake pizza for 15 minutes, then cut in 6 pie-shaped wedges and serve piping hot.

19.8 grams of carbohydrate in entire recipe; if serving 6, each serving contains 3.3 grams of carbohydrate.

London Broil with Boursin

This is one of the easiest recipes in this book. It's become a favorite of many of my friends.

Makes 4 servings

1 5-ounce package French Boursin light cheese with herbs, 78 percent reduced fat
1 2-pound piece London broil, cut from the round
Salt and freshly ground pepper to taste

Bring the Boursin to room temperature by allowing it to stand out of the refrigerator for about 2 hours until very soft. Sprinkle the London broil with salt and pepper to taste. Place meat in a preheated broiler and broil for approximately 5 minutes on each side under very high heat. The outside should be browned and the inside rare for the meat to be tender. Remove meat to a large platter and slice diagonally into very thin slices. Pass the softened Boursin separately as a dipping sauce for the meat.

5.0 grams of carbohydrate in entire recipe; if serving 4, each serving contains 1.3 grains of carbohydrate.

NOTE: You may substitute 4- to 8-ounce boneless steaks grilled to your taste for the London broil.

Soy-Glazed London Broil

Would you have ever thought of making London broil Chinese style?

Makes 3 servings

1 flank steak, weighing about 1½ pounds
2 tablespoons soy sauce, 50 percent reduced salt
2 tablespoons dry sherry or saké
1 tablespoon peanut oil
Few drops Tabasco
1½ cloves fresh garlic, minced
2 slices fresh gingerroot, finely minced

Marinate the steak overnight in a mixture of the soy sauce, sherry, oil, Tabasco, garlic and gingerroot. This can be done in a large bowl or better still in a plastic bag. Turn the meat occasionally in the marinade to flavor all parts. Preheat your broiler for at least 10 minutes then broil the meat 3 inches from the flame for approximately 3 minutes on each side, basting with the marinade. Flank steak must be served rare to keep it from becoming tough. If you don't like rare meat, buy another cut of meat for this recipe. To serve, carve the meat at a diagonal, using a 45° angle, into thin slices. Overlap the slices on a heated serving dish and pour the pan juices over them.

6.0 grams of carbohydrate in entire recipe; if serving 3, each serving contains 2.0 grams of carbohydrate.

Roquefort-Topped Steak

Feeling lazy? Don't want to do more than just broil a steak? This takes only 1 minute more.

Makes 4 servings

2 pounds lean, boneless steak, cut in 4 portions
Salt and freshly ground pepper to taste
Garlic powder
2 ounces French Roquefort cheese
4 teaspoons Chablis or other very dry white wine
15 drops Cognac extract or any good brandy extract
4 teaspoons olive oil

Sprinkle steak to taste with salt, pepper, and garlic powder. Broil to desired state of doneness. While steak is broiling, mix together Roquefort cheese, wine, extract, and oil. When steak is done to taste, top with Roquefort mixture, and broil 1 or 2 minutes longer until topping melts. Remove from broiler and pour pan juices over steak.

1.0 grams of carbohydrate in entire recipe; if serving 4, each serving contains 0.3 grams of carbohydrate.

Steak with Chicken-Liver Sauce

An elegant dinner!

Makes 4 servings

1 tablespoon butter
2 tablespoons extra-virgin olive oil
1 large clove of garlic, minced
2 shallots, minced
½ pound chicken livers
1 bay leaf
½ teaspoon salt
Generous sprinkling of freshly ground black pepper
¼ teaspoon sage
¼ teaspoon thyme
½ cup beef stock (may be made with a bouillon cube)
2 teaspoons dry sherry
½ teaspoon Madras curry powder (page 20)
4 ½-pound lean, boneless beef steaks

Heat the butter and 1 tablespoon of oil in a skillet. Add the garlic, shallots, chicken livers, and bay leaf and sauté 3 minutes over high heat. Add salt, pepper, sage, and thyme and sauté 2 minutes more. Discard bay leaf and place liver mixture in a blender. Add beef stock, sherry, and curry powder and blend until smooth. Keep warm over a very low flame.

Heat the remaining oil until it sizzles, add steaks and brown quickly over high heat to the desired doneness. Place steaks on a serving dish, pour chicken-liver sauce over them, and serve.

8.0 grams of carbohydrate in entire recipe; if serving 4, each serving contains 2.0 grams of carbohydrate.

Steak with Mushroom Sauce

Makes 4 servings

3 tablespoons lemon juice
4 shell steaks, about 8 ounces each
Salt and freshly ground pepper to taste
1 teaspoon bacon drippings
2 tablespoons finely chopped shallots
¼ pound mushrooms, thinly sliced
½ clove garlic, finely minced
½ cup dry red wine
1 teaspoon meat extract, such as Bovril
½ bay leaf
1 teaspoon flour
1 teaspoon butter
1 tablespoon dry red wine
Chopped parsley

Pour lemon juice over steaks and let marinate for about 10 minutes. Drain. Sprinkle with salt and pepper. Heat bacon drippings until lightly browned. Add mushrooms and garlic, and sauté for a few minutes more. Add the wine, meat extract, and bay leaf, bring to a boil, and simmer 5 minutes. Put steaks in the gravy, heat 3 minutes, then place on a preheated platter. Keep warm. Thicken gravy with the flour and butter that have been mixed together and thinned with 1 tablespoon wine. Pour a little gravy over steaks and sprinkle with fresh parsley. Serve remaining gravy on the side.

13.7 grams of carbohydrate in entire recipe; if serving 4, each serving contains 3.4 grams of carbohydrate.

Reprinted from *Annemarie's Personal Cookbook* by Annemarie Huste.

Veal Scallops with Chives and Cheese

Veal and cheese are always a good combination.

Makes 6 servings

2 pounds veal scallops, pounded flat*
Salt and freshly ground pepper to taste
2 tablespoons extra-virgin olive oil
2 teaspoons whipped butter
1 cup dry white wine
½ cup fat-free half-and-half
2 tablespoons chives, fresh, frozen, or freeze-dried
6 ounces Swiss Gruyère cheese (page 18), thinly sliced

Salt and pepper the veal scallops. Heat 2 tablespoons of olive oil in a large skillet, or 2 smaller ones. Add the whipped butter and when melted, sauté veal scallops in a single layer about 5 minutes on each side, or until well browned. Remove to a baking dish large enough to hold the veal in a single layer. Deglaze pan or pans with 1 cup dry white wine, scraping up all browned bits from pan bottom. Cook down until liquid is reduced by half the original volume. Add the half-and-half and chives and heat for 2 minutes more or until sauce thickens. Pour the sauce over the veal, top with sliced cheese, and place under broiler. Broil until the cheese melts.

9.7 grams of carbohydrate in entire recipe; if serving 6, each serving contains 1.6 grams of carbohydrate.

---

*Turkey breast cut for scallopini may be substituted for the veal with equally good results.

Party Veal Scallops

Makes 4 servings

1 pound veal scallops, pounded thin*
1 tablespoon extra-virgin olive oil
1 teaspoon whipped butter
1 cup grated Swiss Gruyère cheese (page 18)
½ cup fat-free half-and-half
2 scant teaspoons Dijon-style mustard
½ cup dry white wine
Salt to taste
Generous amount of freshly ground black pepper

Sauté the veal scallops on both sides in a mixture of the oil and the butter. Meanwhile, combine Gruyère cheese, half-and-half, and mustard. Remove the veal scallops to a heatproof, shallow oven dish. Deglaze the pan used for the scallops with wine, scraping up any browned bits. Boil a few minutes to evaporate all alcohol. Pour the wine over the scallops, top with cheese mixture, and place under the broiler until cheese browns. Serve immediately while hot.

15.9 grams of carbohydrate in entire recipe; if serving 4, each serving contains 4.0 grams of carbohydrate.

---

*Turkey breast cut for scallopini may be substituted for the veal with equally good results.

Veal Chops in Mustard Sauce

One of the more delicious ways of preparing veal chops. Fast, too.

Makes 4 servings

1 tablespoon extra-virgin olive oil
4 thick, lean rib veal chops, each weighing approximately 8 ounces
2 teaspoons softened butter
2 tablespoons wine vinegar
1½ teaspoons Dijon-style mustard
3 tablespoons fat-free half-and-half
2 tablespoons olive oil
½ teaspoon salt
¼ teaspoon freshly ground black pepper
4 tablespoons finely chopped fresh parsley

Heat the oil in a heavy, nonstick skillet. Add the chops to the skillet and cook them over medium heat for approximately 10 minutes on each side or till done. In a tiny saucepan, heat the next 7 ingredients together, stirring frequently. Do not boil the mixture. When the chops are cooked, remove them to a heated platter. Pour off any excess fat that may have accumulated in the skillet and add the mustard mixture to the pan. Heat over a low flame to combine the mustard mixture with the pan juices. Pour the sauce over the chops and garnish with chopped parsley.

6.5 grams of carbohydrate in entire recipe; if serving 4, each serving contains 1.6 grams of carbohydrate.

Grilled Lamb Chops or Lamb Steaks with Mint Pesto

Makes 4 servings

Mint Pesto

2½ cups fresh mint leaves, washed and dried
2 large cloves fresh garlic
2 tablespoons pine nuts
4 tablespoons extra-virgin olive oil
A few drops fresh lemon juice
Salt and freshly ground pepper to taste

With the food processor running, chop the garlic. Stop the food processor. Add the mint leaves and the pine nuts and continue chopping. Slowly add the oil and lemon juice and process until smooth. Season to taste with salt and pepper and set aside.

Grilled Lamb

4 lamb steaks or 4 shoulder lamb chops or 8 rib or loin lamb chops
Garlic powder or fresh garlic put through a press
Poissonnade (This is a French herb mixture for fish, which I feel balances out the stronger taste of lamb better than the other blend of herbs de Provence.)
Salt and freshly ground pepper to taste

Trim the fat from the lamb steaks or chops, or have your butcher do this for you. If the lamb steaks are very lean, brush them with a little extra-virgin olive oil. The chops usually will not need this. Place the lamb in a foil broiling pan with ridges or in a grill pan or on an electric grill. (In the wintertime, I'll use the broiler part of my oven, but in the warmer weather, I'll use my grill pan on top of the stove or my electric grill so I don't heat up the house. My electric grill has plates that come off for washing, making them easier to clean.) Season both sides of the lamb lightly with the garlic (or garlic powder, in an emergency) and crush the poissonnade with your fingers, as you sprinkle it on the steak. Grill to your taste and then add salt and freshly ground pepper. I like lamb left pink, French style, rather than well done. Try it that way; the worst that can happen is that you don't like it, in which case you can grill it a little longer. You might be in for a pleasant surprise. Serve at once on heated plates with the Mint Pesto on the side.

8.4 grams of carbohydrate in entire recipe; makes 4 servings, each serving containing 2.1 grams of carbohydrate.

Lamb Shish Kebab

This recipe was given to me by one of the women I once worked with. I can no longer remember her name, but I've never forgotten her delicious recipe.

Makes 2 servings

¼ cup olive oil
¼ cup dry white wine
2 tablespoons grated onion
½ teaspoon garlic powder
½ teaspoon salt
½ teaspoon freshly ground black pepper
1 teaspoon caraway seeds
1 teaspoon oregano
1 pound lean, boneless lamb
1 medium green pepper, cut in 8 pieces
6 tiny, white onions, parboiled for 10 minutes
1 small tomato, quartered
4 medium mushroom caps

Combine the oil, wine, onion, garlic powder, salt, pepper, caraway seeds, and oregano in a bowl. Cut the lamb into 1½-inch cubes and add to the marinade. Stir the lamb in the marinade until it is thoroughly coated. Marinate the meat at least 24 hours or longer, if you prefer, turning the cubes occasionally. Thread the meat on skewers, alternating with the green pepper, white onions, tomato, and mushroom caps. Broil under a high flame, turning the skewers until the meat is brown on all sides but still pink inside. Lamb tastes better when it is not too well done. Baste occasionally with the marinade while broiling. Serve hot.

22.2 grams of carbohydrate in entire recipe; if serving 2, each serving contains 11.1 grams of carbohydrate.

Sautéed Calf's Liver

Makes 4 servings

30 grams (¼ cup, unsifted) full-fat soy flour
½ teaspoon salt
2 dashes garlic powder
2 dashes ground celery seed
¼ teaspoon freshly ground black pepper
2 pounds calf's liver, sliced ⅜–½ inch thick
1 tablespoon whipped butter and 3 tablespoons extra-virgin olive oil
1 cup dry white wine
2 tablespoons chopped fresh chives
Parsley for garnish

Combine the soy flour with the salt, garlic powder, onion powder, celery seed, and black pepper. Dredge the liver in seasoned soy flour and shake off excess flour. Heat the butter and oil in a large, heavy skillet, arrange the liver in a single layer, and sauté 2 to 3 minutes, regulating the flame so the butter mixture is always very hot but not burning. Turn liver and sauté for 1 or 2 minutes more. The liver is done when it is just a pale pink inside. Remove to a hot platter and add the wine to the skillet. Over a high flame, deglaze the pans, scraping up any browned bits. Cook briefly until the alcohol smell has completely disappeared. Add chopped chives and cook another minute. Pour the sauce over the liver, decorate platter with parsley sprigs, and serve hot.

47.0 grams of carbohydrate in entire recipe; if serving 4, each serving contains 12.0 grams of carbohydrate.

NOTE: When purchasing the liver, ask the butcher to remove the surrounding filament from each slice of liver. If filament is left on, the liver will curl as it cooks.

V.

Fish: Gifts from the Sea

Broiled Bluefish with Bacon   145
Mustard-Flavored Spanish Mackerel   146
Grilled Salmon Steaks with Anchovy Butter   147
Shad en Papillote   148
Sole Cordon Bleu   149
Fillet of Sole with Parmesan Cheese   150
Scampi   150
Curried Shrimp Salad   152
Broiled Lobster Tails   152
Seafood Kebabs   153
Sesame-Crusted Tuna Fish   154

Fish: Gifts from the Sea

I think the reason most people don't like fish is that the fish we get in supermarkets is not fresh enough. When really fresh, fish has neither a fishy smell nor a fishy taste. It is delicate and delicious! Things to look for when buying fresh fish are bright, sparkling eyes, flesh that springs back when pressed, and no fishy smell.

Broiled Bluefish with Bacon

The bacon on this may even please a fish-hater.

Makes 2 servings

1 2¼–2½-pound bluefish, filleted (1 pound of fillets)
Garlic powder
Freshly ground pepper
2 thick slices bacon
Minced parsley
Lemon slices

Make individual trays for each serving out of double-weight aluminum foil because it is very difficult to remove the fish without ruining the way it looks. Place each serving of fish on its own tray and sprinkle lightly with garlic powder and pepper. Place a strip of bacon on each piece and broil until fish flakes easily when tested with a fork, basting frequently with bacon drippings. If bacon gets crisp before fish is ready, remove to a warm platter and keep warm.

When the fish tests done, remove it, foil and all, to a serving platter. Sprinkle each serving with freshly minced parsley, place a lemon slice alongside, and top with a crisp slice of bacon. Serve fish hot in its own tray. Coleslaw makes a nice accompaniment.

1.9 grams of carbohydrate in entire recipe; if serving 2, each serving contains 1.0 grams of carbohydrate.

Mustard-Flavored Spanish Mackerel

Makes 4 servings

3 tablespoons extra-virgin olive oil
1 tablespoon whipped butter
2 tablespoons Dijon-style mustard
¼ cup fresh lemon juice
Spanish mackerel fillets weighing about 2 pounds
Salt and freshly ground black pepper to taste
2 tablespoons fresh dill, finely chopped

Melt the butter and oil in a tiny saucepan. Mix in the mustard and the lemon juice. Wash and dry the fillets, then sprinkle them to taste with salt and freshly ground black pepper. Arrange the fillets on aluminum foil, skin side down. Baste the fish with approximately ½ of the mustard-butter mixture and broil it for a few minutes. Baste the fish with the remaining mustard-butter and continue to broil until the fish flakes easily when tested with a fork. Sprinkle with the chopped dill and serve immediately.

8.2 grams of carbohydrate in entire recipe; if serving 4, each serving contains 2.1 grams of carbohydrate.

Grilled Salmon Steaks with Anchovy Butter

Anchovy butter makes a delicious accent for grilled salmon.

Makes 4 servings

2 tablespoons extra-virgin olive oil
1 teaspoon dried tarragon or 1 tablespoon fresh tarragon, if available
4 8-ounce fresh salmon steaks or fillets of salmon
Salt and freshly ground pepper to taste (Be aware that anchovy butter is salty, so go easy on any salt you add.)
4 tablespoons whipped butter, softened
2 teaspoons anchovy paste

Warm 2 tablespoons of the oil and add the tarragon to it. Brush salmon steaks or fillets with half of the tarragon-oil mixture, then sprinkle very lightly with salt and pepper. Place in a preheated broiler and broil until one side is golden brown. If using salmon steaks, turn the fish, brush with the remaining tarragon-oil mixture, and broil second side down until it is golden brown. If using salmon fillets, do not turn them. The fish should flake easily when tested with a fork.

While the salmon is broiling, make anchovy butter by creaming together the softened butter with the anchovy paste. Shape the mixture into pats, circles, or rosettes and refrigerate until the salmon is ready. Remove the salmon to a warm platter and top each piece with anchovy butter.

1.8 grams of carbohydrate in entire recipe; if serving 4, each serving contains 0.5 grams of carbohydrate.

Shad en Papillote

This is the nicest way I've ever found to prepare fish.

Makes 4 servings

2 pounds shad fillets, cut in 4 pieces
4 teaspoons dry white wine
4 tablespoons fat-free half-and-half
Garlic powder
Salt and freshly ground pepper to taste
4 tablespoons grated Parmesan cheese
Lemon wedges
Parsley for garnish

Preheat oven to 425° F. Make 4 casings of aluminum foil large enough to hold each piece of fish with room to make a double fold at the edges. The foil may be cut like a large folded heart or a folded rectangle. (To make a heart, take each piece of aluminum foil, fold it in half to double it, and cut out a large heart that is joined at the bottom where you have folded it.)

Place 1 shad fillet piece in the center of each foil casing and sprinkle with a teaspoon of wine. Add 1 tablespoon of half-and-half to each fillet, then sprinkle lightly with garlic powder, salt, pepper, and 1 tablespoon of Parmesan cheese. Seal the foil packages tightly by folding both edges together twice. Bake in the preheated oven for 20 minutes, at which time the fish should be done, flaking easily when tested with a fork. Serve in the foil. It looks very impressive, particularly if you have made the hearts. Decorate each plate with lemon wedges and fresh parsley.

6.8 grams of carbohydrate in entire recipe; if serving 4, each serving contains 1.7 grams of carbohydrate.

NOTE: If shad is not available, try this method with other white-meat fish.

Sole Cordon Bleu

Makes 4 servings

4 fillets of sole, 8 ounces each
½ cup dry white wine
Salt and freshly ground pepper to taste
Garlic powder
Dried dill weed (you can use fresh if available)
2 teaspoons butter and 2 teaspoons extra-virgin olive oil
¼ pound boiled ham, cut into 4 slices
¼ pound Swiss cheese, preferably imported, cut into
   4 slices
Parsley for garnish

Wash and dry fillets, and arrange them in a shallow baking dish. Pour 1 tablespoon of wine over each fillet, then salt and pepper, and sprinkle lightly with garlic powder and dill. Dot with 2 teaspoons of the butter mixture. Broil until fish just begins to acquire color (if browned, it will get too dry). With a pancake turner, turn the fillets over carefully without breaking them. Pour 1 tablespoon of remaining wine over each piece, then sprinkle again lightly with salt, pepper, garlic powder, and dill. Dot with the remaining butter mixture and broil until golden. Baste continually during the broiling on both sides with the wine drippings in the pan.

When fish is golden, cover each fillet with a ham slice and broil 1 or 2 minutes to warm the ham. Then cover each with a cheese slice and allow to broil until cheese melts (about 2 minutes more). Remove fish to warmed plates and pour any pan drippings over it. Garnish with sprigs of fresh parsley.

3.2 grams of carbohydrate in entire recipe; if serving 4, each serving contains 0.8 grams of carbohydrate.

Fillet of Sole with Parmesan Cheese

Would you like a quick fish meal?

Serves 4

4 8-ounce fillets of sole
1 teaspoon salt
¼ teaspoon freshly ground black pepper
Dash of garlic powder
3 tablespoons extra-virgin olive oil
1 tablespoon whipped butter
½ cup grated Parmesan cheese
¼ cup bottled clam juice

Wash and dry the fillets. Season to taste with salt, garlic powder, and pepper. Heat 2 tablespoons of the oil in a nonstick skillet and sauté the fish in it until golden brown on both sides. Sprinkle with cheese and the clam juice. Dot with the remaining butter and oil. Cover the pan and cook over low heat for another 5 minutes.

3.2 grams of carbohydrate in entire recipe; if serving 4, each serving contains 0.8 grams of carbohydrate.

Scampi

Italy's gift to the diet world!

Makes 6 appetizer servings or 3 main dish servings

1½ pounds very large fresh shrimp in the shell
2 tablespoons whipped butter, melted
4 tablespoons extra-virgin olive oil
2 large or 4 small cloves garlic, finely minced
1 teaspoon salt
Freshly ground black pepper
4 tablespoons finely chopped parsley
Lemon wedges

Shell the shrimp, or have it done, making sure the last quarter inch of shell (the tail) is left on. Slit the shrimp down the back and lift out black veins. Wash shrimp with cold water and dry with paper towels.

Combine the melted butter, olive oil, garlic, salt, and pepper and marinate the shrimp in this mixture 1 to 2 hours. (Don't worry if the butter coagulates as it gets cold; it will melt again during broiling.)

Preheat the broiler. Place shrimp in a shallow, flameproof baking dish or in individual dishes and pour the marinade over it. Broil the shrimp 3 to 4 inches from the heat for 5 minutes. Turn them over and broil 5 to 10 minutes more until lightly browned and firm to the touch. Baste frequently while broiling. (Do not overcook!) Sprinkle with minced parsley and garnish with lemon wedges. Serve very hot.

8.3 grams of carbohydrate in entire recipe if serving 6 as an appetizer, each serving contains 1.4 grams of carbohydrate; if serving 3 as a main dish, each serving contains 2.8 grams of carbohydrate.

Curried Shrimp Salad

An interesting version of shrimp salad.

Makes 4 servings

2 cups cooked, cleaned tiny shrimp
1 cup diced celery
½ cup sugarless mayonnaise
1½–2 teaspoons Madras curry powder (page 20)
Dash of garlic powder
Salt and freshly ground pepper to taste
Cantaloupe wedges

If only large shrimp are available, dice them. Mix together the cooked shrimp, celery, mayonnaise, curry powder, garlic powder, salt, and pepper. Chill until serving time. To serve, arrange a scoop of shrimp salad on a lettuce leaf and garnish with a wedge of cantaloupe.

10.8 grams of carbohydrate in entire recipe; if serving 4, each serving contains 2.7 grams of carbohydrate.

Broiled Lobster Tails

An expensive treat, but an absolutely delicious dinner.

Makes 4 servings

4 large lobster tails, about 12 ounces each
2 tablespoons whipped butter
5 tablespoons extra-virgin olive oil
2 teaspoons chopped fresh basil
½ teaspoon chopped fresh rosemary

Fish: Gifts from the Sea 153

½ teaspoon chopped fresh thyme
1 large lemon, cut into 4 wedges

Have the fishmonger split the lobster tails down the middle and clean them. Warm the butter and oil together. Brush the lobster tails with a little of the oil-butter mixture and broil for 12 to 18 minutes, brushing occasionally with the oil-butter mixture. When done, the tails will be golden brown and the lobster meat will come away from the shell. (Do not overcook!)

While the tails are cooking, add the herbs to the oil-butter mixture and allow to sit and absorb flavor while the lobster tails broil. When they are finished, divide the herb butter into 4 small dishes. Serve a dish of the herb butter for dipping the lobster meat on the same plate as you serve the lobster tail. Add a lemon wedge to the plate so that the lemon juice may be squeezed into the butter mixture.

8.0 grams of carbohydrate in entire recipe; if serving 4, each serving contains 2.0 grams of carbohydrate.

Seafood Kebabs

Makes 2–3 servings

4 tablespoons olive oil
2 tablespoons dry vermouth
Salt and freshly ground pepper to taste
6 ounces fresh lobster meat, cut into 1½-inch cubes
6 ounces fresh scallops, halved crosswise
6 ounces fresh shrimp, cleaned and deveined (8 ounces before cleaning)
8 medium-size fresh mushroom caps
1 medium tomato, cut in eighths
1 green pepper, cut in eighths
8 tiny white onions, parboiled 10 minutes

Mix together in a large bowl the oil, vermouth, salt and pepper. Place the lobster meat, scallops, and shrimp in the oil mixture and stir to coat thoroughly. Cover with aluminum foil and refrigerate overnight.

Preheat the broiler for 15 minutes. Arrange the seafood on skewers, alternating the seafood with the vegetables. Broil for 12 to 18 minutes, depending on your broiler, until done, basting frequently with the marinade. Do not overcook.

43.0 grams of carbohydrate in entire recipe; if serving 3, each serving contains 14.3 grams of carbohydrate.

Sesame-Crusted Tuna Fish

If you have never tasted fresh tuna, you're in for a treat. I love tuna fish in any form, fresh or canned. In fact, tuna fish salad on toast is my nursery food if I'm very upset and can't eat. I loved it as a child and would even ask my mother if I could have it for my breakfast. Fortunately, my mother was not difficult about food and wanted us to enjoy our meals. She never forced us to eat anything we didn't like and usually made us our favorite things. Be aware that fresh tuna does not taste good if it's well done. It should be charred on the outside and rare on the inside.

Makes 4 servings

4 fresh tuna fish steaks, about 8 ounces each, preferably cut 1¼ to 1½ inches thick (This helps it grill rare on the inside while the outside is crisped.)
1 tablespoon and 1 teaspoon soy sauce, 50 percent reduced salt
1 tablespoon and 1 teaspoon extra-virgin olive oil
2 teaspoons medium dry sherry (I use an Amontillado)
A few dashes of garlic powder or a clove of crushed garlic
1 extra tablespoon extra-virgin olive oil
60 grams roasted sesame seeds (approximately ¼ cup and 1 teaspoon)

Wash and dry the tuna steaks. With a fork or miniwhisk, beat together the soy sauce, oil, sherry, and garlic powder. Brush the mixture on the tuna steaks, then dredge them or generously sprinkle them with the sesame seeds. Brush the broiler pan, grill pan, or electric grill plates with the extra olive oil and preheat to very hot. Grill the tuna steaks for 2 to 3 minutes on each side for medium rare. Serve the tuna steaks with green wasabi (easily made by mixing green wasabi powder from the can with water to make a paste) and with sugar-free sweet pickled ginger. (I found the sugar-free ginger and the wasabi powder at my local greengrocer. They can also be found in Asian markets or in the Asian section of your local supermarket.)

10.8 grams of carbohydrate in entire recipe; makes 4 servings, each serving containing 2.7 grams of carbohydrate.

Basic Flavoring Recipe for Fish

This works well for almost any fish, be it tuna, salmon, swordfish, rainbow trout, Chilean sea bass, etc., whether you are grilling the fish, microwaving the fish (really a form of steaming), or using a foil casing. I've tried it on almost every fish; when flavored this way it's very fast and always tastes good.

Extra-virgin olive oil
Garlic powder (or fresh; powder is more subtle)
Poissonnade (see page 16)
White wine or dry vermouth (optional)
Salt and freshly ground pepper to taste
Lemon wedges

Brush fish with the olive oil, then spoon 1 to 2 tablespoons of white wine or vermouth over each piece. Sprinkle fish with garlic powder, then with poissonnade. Add salt and pepper to taste and serve with lemon wedges.

VI.

Chicken: A Dieter's Best Friend

Broiled Chicken with Shallot Butter   159
Mustard-Broiled Chicken   160
Chicken in Blue Cheese Sauce   161
Broiled Chicken aux Fines Herbes   162
Chicken with Cream and Herbs   163
Soy-Glazed Chicken Breasts   164
Curried Chicken Breasts   165
Curried Chicken Salad   166
Chicken Liver Sauté   166
Chicken with Pesto and Ricotta   167
Baked Skinless and Boneless Chicken Breasts   168
Broiled Chicken with Pesto   168
Apricot-Glazed Turkey London Broil   169
Glazed Rock Cornish Hens   170
Party Cornish Hens   172

Chicken: A Dieter's Best Friend

Chicken is excellent for low-carbohydrate diets because not only is it low in carbohydrates and calories, it is also one of our most versatile foods. It is relatively inexpensive, combines well with many seasonings, and is delicious in salads, dressed up in its Sunday best, or just simply roasted or broiled with no trimmings!

Broiled Chicken with Shallot Butter

A delicate way of preparing chicken and a favorite of anyone who has tried it.

Makes 2 servings

2 chicken breasts (about 1 pound each), halved
6 tablespoons minced shallots
1 tablespoon softened whipped butter
3 tablespoons extra-virgin olive oil*
Salt and freshly ground pepper to taste

Let the butter stand out for 10 to 15 minutes to soften a little. Combine the minced shallots with the softened butter and oil.* Divide the shallot butter into 4 equal parts and push one part under the skin of each quarter of chicken. Sprinkle the chicken breasts with salt and freshly ground black pepper to taste. Place the chicken breasts, skin side down, in a broiling pan. Broil the chicken breasts for 13 to 15 minutes. Turn the breasts over, skin side up, and broil them for 13 to 15 minutes more or till done. Baste them frequently with the shallot-flavored butter that has seeped out from under the skin. Remove to a heated serving platter and pour the shallot-flavored drippings over the chicken breasts.

7.2 grams of carbohydrate in entire recipe; if serving 2, each serving contains 3.6 grams of carbohydrate.

*NOTE: Partially freeze the butter, oil, and shallot mixture. This is a bit tricky but is necessary to stiffen the oil so it can be put under the skin. I admit being proud to have thought of this.

Mustard-Broiled Chicken

Here's a chicken recipe for the mustard lovers.

Makes 4 servings

4 whole chicken breasts (about 1 pound each), halved
½ cup Italian olive oil
3 tablespoons brown mustard
Salt and freshly ground pepper to taste
Lemon wedges

Arrange the chicken breasts, skin side down, on aluminum foil or on a broiling pan. Add the oil to the mustard slowly, beating with a fork to the consistency of mayonnaise. Brush the underside of chicken breasts with about a third of the mustard mixture. Broil 13 to 15 minutes. Turn chicken skin side up, spread with remaining mustard mixture, and broil 13 to 15 minutes more, basting frequently with pan drippings. Sprinkle with salt and freshly ground pepper to taste and serve a lemon wedge alongside each portion of chicken.

4.5 grams of carbohydrate in entire recipe; if serving 4, each serving contains 1.1 grams of carbohydrate.

Chicken in Blue Cheese Sauce

An unusual combination of flavors that blend well together. The liquid smoke adds a high note.

Makes 4 servings

1 cup cottage cheese
2 ounces blue cheese
¼ cup chopped parsley
1 tablespoon softened whipped butter
3 tablespoons extra-virgin olive oil
½ teaspoon salt
1 small clove garlic, crushed
¼ cup cold water
2 teaspoons liquid smoke
4 whole chicken breasts (about 1 pound each), halved

Combine cottage cheese, blue cheese, parsley, butter, oil, salt, garlic, water, and liquid smoke in a blender until smooth. This will make a lovely green-colored sauce.

Wash and dry chicken breasts. Arrange them skin side down on heavy duty aluminum foil or on a broiling pan. Spread about a third of the cheese mixture over the chicken and broil 13 to 15 minutes. Turn chicken breasts skin side up and spread remaining cheese mixture on the skin. Broil another 13 to 15 minutes, basting occasionally with pan drippings. Serve hot.

8.6 grams of carbohydrate in entire recipe; if serving 4, each serving contains 2.2 grams of carbohydrate.

Broiled Chicken aux Fines Herbes

A fines herbes *mixture is just as good with chicken as it is with eggs.*

Makes 4 servings

2 tablespoons softened butter
6 tablespoons extra-virgin olive oil
½ cup chopped chives, fresh or frozen
½ cup chopped fresh parsley
2 teaspoons dried tarragon
2 cloves garlic, crushed
4 whole chicken breasts (about 1 pound each), halved
Salt and freshly ground pepper to taste

Combine butter and oil, chives, parsley, tarragon, and garlic and partially freeze.* Wash and dry chicken breasts, then salt and pepper them. Divide butter mixture into 8 equal parts. Stuff 1 part under the skin of each chicken breast, spreading it throughout the skin. Place chicken breasts skin side down on aluminum foil or on a broiling pan and broil 13 to 15 minutes. Turn skin side up and broil 13 to 15 minutes more, basting frequently with the pan drippings. Serve hot with the pan drippings poured over the chicken.

3.4 grams of carbohydrate in entire recipe; if serving 4, each serving contains 0.9 grams of carbohydrate.

*NOTE: Partially freezing the butter-oil herb mixture is a bit tricky, but is necessary to stiffen the oil so it can be put under the skin.

Chicken with Cream and Herbs

The nutmeg in this recipe adds the high note.

Makes 4 servings

3 whole chicken breasts (about 1 pound each), halved
Salt and freshly ground pepper to taste
2 teaspoons whipped butter
4 teaspoons extra-virgin olive oil
3 tablespoons minced shallots
6 tablespoons dry white wine or dry vermouth
6 tablespoons dry sherry
6 tablespoons chicken broth
6 tablespoons fat-free half-and-half
2 egg yolks
2 tablespoons minced parsley
2 tablespoons minced chives
Generous dash of freshly ground nutmeg

Wash and dry chicken breasts and sprinkle with salt and pepper. Heat butter and oil together in a large skillet. (The oil will keep the butter from burning.) Sauté the shallots lightly, then add chicken breasts, and brown until tender. Remove to a warm platter and pour off excess fat from the pan.

Mix together the wine, sherry, and chicken broth. Deglaze the pan with this mixture, scraping up any browned bits. Cook the liquid for a few minutes until the alcohol smell evaporates. Beat the egg yolks with the half-and-half and add to the pan, stirring constantly until heated (do not allow to boil). Add parsley, chives, and a dash of nutmeg to the sauce. To serve, spoon the sauce over the chicken breasts and serve hot.

13.6 grams of carbohydrate in entire recipe; if serving 4, each serving contains 3.4 grams of carbohydrate.

Soy-Glazed Chicken Breasts

Serves 3

3 whole chicken breasts (about 1 pound each), halved
Salt and freshly ground pepper to taste
Garlic powder
3 tablespoons soy sauce, 50 percent reduced salt
⅓ cup water
1–2 tablespoons minced fresh gingerroot
3 tablespoons sugar-free orange marmalade

Halve the chicken breasts, then wash and dry them. Sprinkle lightly with salt, pepper, and garlic powder. Arrange in broiling pan or on aluminum foil skin side down.

Combine soy sauce, water, and gingerroot. Baste the chicken with this mixture, and broil 13 to 15 minutes. Turn chicken skin side up, cover with remaining soy sauce mixture, and broil 13 to 15 minutes longer, basting frequently with pan drippings. When chicken is almost done, spread with the marmalade and broil 2 to 3 minutes longer. To serve, pour a little of the soy mixture from the pan on the chicken.

23.4 grams of carbohydrate in entire recipe; makes 3 servings, each serving containing 7.8 grams of carbohydrate.

Curried Chicken Breasts

Makes 4 servings

8 *suprêmes* (See NOTE)
1 teaspoon lemon juice
1 teaspoon salt
White pepper
1 tablespoon whipped butter
3 tablespoons extra-virgin olive oil
½ cup chicken stock
½ cup dry white wine
½ cup fat-free half-and-half
¾–1 teaspoon curry powder

Preheat oven to 400° F. Rub the *suprêmes* with lemon juice, and sprinkle with salt and pepper. In 2 large ovenproof skillets or casseroles, heat the butter until foamy and then add the oil. Roll the *suprêmes* in the hot butter-oil mixture, putting 4 in each skillet. Cover each skillet with buttered waxed paper, cut to fit, and a regular cover. Place in preheated oven and cook 7 to 8 minutes or until chicken feels firm and slightly springy when tested with your finger. Remove to a hot serving platter, leaving butter in the pans. Keep warm.

Add chicken broth and wine to the skillets, and boil over a high flame until the liquid becomes slightly syrupy. Add the half-and-half and curry powder and cook for another minute or 2 until slightly thickened. Pour the sauce over the *suprêmes* and serve hot.

13.7 grams of carbohydrate in entire recipe; if serving 4, each serving contains 3.4 grams of carbohydrate.

NOTE: To quote Julia Child, "Breast of chicken, when it is removed raw from one side of the bird in a skinless, boneless piece, is called a *'suprême.'* Each chicken possesses two of them."

Curried Chicken Salad

Curry powder makes an interesting and delicious variation for chicken salad.

Makes 6 servings

3 cups cooked chicken, diced
2 cups diced celery
1 cup sugarless mayonnaise
2–3 teaspoons curry powder
Dash of garlic powder
Cantaloupe wedges

Combine diced chicken and diced celery. Mix in the mayonnaise. Add 2 or 3 teaspoons of curry powder, depending on the degree of spiciness you like, and a dash of garlic powder. Mix all ingredients thoroughly and serve scoops of the chicken salad on lettuce leaves. Cantaloupe wedges served on the side make a good taste contrast.

15.6 grams of carbohydrate in entire recipe; if serving 6, each serving contains 2.6 grams of carbohydrate.

Chicken Liver Sauté

Even people who don't like liver frequently like chicken livers.

Makes 4 servings

2 slices bacon, cut into small pieces
1 small onion, chopped
1 tablespoon extra-virgin olive oil
1 pound chicken livers
½ cup sliced mushrooms

3 tablespoons Chablis or similar dry white wine
¼ teaspoon sage (a pinch more if desired)
Salt and freshly ground pepper to taste

Sauté the bacon and onion together. Add oil, chicken livers, and mushrooms and cook, stirring frequently, until the livers are browned but pink inside. Add the wine, sage, salt and pepper and cook 2 minutes longer. Serve piping hot as an appetizer or light luncheon dish or use as a filling for a French omelet.

23.1 grams of carbohydrate in entire recipe; if serving 4, each serving contains 5.8 grams of carbohydrate.

Chicken with Pesto and Ricotta

The idea for this recipe came from Joyce Goldstein, owner/chef of Square One, a restaurant in San Francisco. If I get to San Francisco, I would love to eat in her restaurant. This recipe is another excuse to eat Pesto Sauce.

Makes 4 servings

4 chicken breasts, with skin and bone, halved
½ cup ricotta, part-skim variety
2 tablespoons Pesto Sauce (page 262)

Wash and dry the chicken breasts. Combine the ricotta and Pesto Sauce and divide it into 8 equal parts. Stuff one part under the skin of each half of chicken breast, spreading it throughout the skin. Place chicken breasts skin side down on a broiling pan and broil 13 to 15 minutes. Turn the chicken skin side up and broil 13 to 15 minutes more, basting frequently with the pan drippings. The juices should run clear; that tells you the chicken is fully cooked. Serve hot with the drippings poured over the chicken.

6.0 grams of carbohydrate in entire recipe; if serving 4, each serving contains 1.5 grams of carbohydrate.

Baked Skinless and Boneless Chicken Breasts

Here we're using the same ricotta and pesto mixture as in the previous recipe, but the chicken has no skin for those who prefer it that way. More pesto again! I hope that you like pesto as much as I do.

Makes 4 servings

4 skinless, boneless chicken breasts, halved
½ cup ricotta, part-skim variety
2 tablespoons Pesto Sauce (page 262)
Olive oil spray

Preheat oven to 350° F. Wash and dry the chicken breasts. Spray a baking dish with olive oil spray. Combine the ricotta and Pesto Sauce. Place chicken breasts in the prepared baking dish and top with the ricotta and pesto mixture. Bake for approximately 30 to 35 minutes or until done.

6.0 grams of carbohydrate in entire recipe; if serving 4, each serving contains 1.5 grams of carbohydrate.

Broiled Chicken with Pesto

Since I made pesto sauce, I had fun trying it in different ways.

Makes 4 servings

4 whole chicken breasts, with skin and bone, halved
½ cup Pesto Sauce (page 262)

Semi-freeze the Pesto Sauce to make it firmer to handle. Wash and dry the chicken breasts. Divide the Pesto Sauce into 8 equal parts. Push one part under the skin of each piece of chicken breast, spreading it throughout the skin. Place the chicken on a broiling pan, skin side down. Broil 13 to 15 minutes, then turn the chicken skin side up and broil for 13 to 15 minutes more, basting frequently with the pan drippings. The juices should run clear; that tells you that the chicken is fully cooked. Serve hot with the pan drippings poured over the chicken.

8.0 grams of carbohydrate in entire recipe; if serving 4, each serving contains 2.0 grams of carbohydrate.

Apricot-Glazed Turkey London Broil

The idea for this recipe originated from my recipe for Glazed Rock Cornish Hens (page 170), which were always a favorite of mine. Yes, even cookbook authors have their favorite recipes.

Makes 4 servings

½ boneless turkey breast, skin removed, weighing
   approximately 1½ pounds
1 tablespoon whipped butter
3 tablespoons extra-virgin olive oil
4 tablespoons chopped chives, fresh or frozen
1 teaspoon dried rosemary, crushed
1 tablespoon fresh lemon juice
¼ cup sugar-free apricot jam
Granulated artificial sweetener equal to 8 teaspoons sugar*

---

*Whether or not you need to add sweetener to the apricot jam will depend on the brand of jam that you are using. Taste it! If it doesn't taste sweet enough to you, add the sweetener to it. It's impossible for me to cover all the brands that are currently on the market now or that may come out in the future. I tried all the brands that were currently available and found that some needed extra sweetener and some did not. Again, taste the apricot jam.

Wash and dry the turkey breast. Warm the butter and oil together. Remove from the heat and add the chives, rosemary, and lemon juice. Place the turkey breast in a broiling pan or in a grill pan or on an electric grill. (In the wintertime, I'll use the broiler that's part of my stove, but in the warmer weather, I'll use my grill pan or my electric grill so I don't heat up the house. My electric grill has ridged plates that come off for washing, making them easier to clean.) Brush with the butter, oil, and herb mixture. Grill to an internal temperature of 170° F. when tested at the thickest part. This will take about 20 minutes on each side. Test the turkey breast; you should not eat poultry that is not cooked thoroughly.

While grilling, continue to baste with the herb mixture. When the turkey breast is almost ready, warm the apricot jam; remove from the heat and add the sweetener to it. When the turkey is almost done, brush it evenly on all sides with the apricot jam and continue grilling until it is nicely glazed. Serve hot when freshly made but be aware that this is great cold the next day if you have any leftovers.

21.6 grams of carbohydrate in entire recipe; if serving 4, each serving contains 5.4 grams of carbohydrate.

NOTE: My market sells half of a skinless, boneless turkey breast as turkey London broil. That's how I learned about it. Most markets will be happy to prepare it that way for you if you ask. You may even give them an idea for a new way of selling turkey.

Glazed Rock Cornish Hens

The inspiration for these hens came from a Sunset cookbook and they make one of the most impressive meals you can serve.

Makes 6 to 8 servings

Chicken: A Dieter's Best Friend

4 fresh Rock Cornish game hens, thawed, each weighing about 1½ to 2 pounds (Use frozen if fresh are not available.)
Salt and freshly ground pepper to taste
2 tablespoons whipped butter
6 tablespoons extra-virgin olive oil
4 tablespoons chopped chives, fresh or frozen
1 teaspoon dried rosemary, crushed
2 tablespoons lemon juice
¼ cup dietetic apricot jam
Granulated artificial sweetener equal to 8 teaspoons sugar*

Preheat oven to 350° F. Wash the hens thoroughly, then dry inside and outside with paper towels. Sprinkle the skin and cavities with salt and pepper.

Warm the butter and oil. Remove from the heat, and add the chives and rosemary. Place about 1 tablespoon of the melted butter mixture inside each hen. Close the hens with small metal skewers or toothpicks. Tie the legs together with clean string. Add the lemon juice to the remaining butter mixture. Place hens in a roasting pan, breast side up. Baste them with the herb-flavored butter and roast them for about 1 hour, turning the hens occasionally and basting with the herb-flavored butter. After 1 hour, raise the oven temperature to 575° F. to brown and crispen the skin.

Warm the apricot jam. Remove from the heat and add the sweetener to it. When the hens are almost done, brush them evenly with the jam and continue roasting them until nicely glazed. Remove the string and serve hot.

22.8 grams of carbohydrate in entire recipe; if serving 4, each serving contains 5.7 grams of carbohydrate.

*See suggestion on page 169 regarding sweetening of jam.

Party Cornish Hens

Makes 6 to 8 servings

Four 1½-pound Rock Cornish hens
¼ cup Japanese soy sauce, 50 percent reduced salt
¼ cup dry sherry
¼ cup peanut oil
1 small clove garlic, minced

Preheat the oven to 350° F. Wash and dry the hens thoroughly, then arrange them in a roasting pan. Mix together the soy sauce, sherry, oil, and garlic. Brush the hens with the soy sauce mixture. Use any remaining sauce to baste the hens as they cook. Roast 1 hour in preheated oven, then turn the heat up to 550° F. for 10 to 15 minutes more to brown the hens. Remove from the heat and serve immediately.

6.6 grams of carbohydrate in entire recipe; if serving 8, each serving contains 0.8 grams of carbohydrate.

VII.

Eggs and Egg Dishes: Thanks to the Chickens

Scrambled Eggs 175
Omelets Aplenty 177
Soufflés 188

Eggs and Egg Dishes: Thanks to the Chickens

This chapter could almost have been called "Omelets Aplenty." Eggs are delicious by themselves when well prepared, but omelets are the most delicious of all. Give an omelet an interesting filling and it can be used for breakfast, lunch, or dinner.

Scrambled Eggs

Cheddar Scrambled Eggs

Eggs and cheese are just meant for each other.

Serves 1

2 eggs
1 ounce very sharp white Cheddar cheese, grated
1 teaspoon whipped butter
1 teaspoon very light olive oil
Parsley for garnish
Freshly ground black pepper to taste

Break eggs into a bowl and beat thoroughly with a wire whisk. Add grated cheese to eggs. Melt butter and oil in a nonstick skillet and add egg mixture, stirring frequently to allow all uncooked egg to reach the bottom of the pan. Use a medium-low flame. As eggs set, cheese will begin to melt, streaking the eggs with melted cheese. Cook until you see there are no more separate pieces of cheese, then remove to a warm plate. Garnish with chopped parsley and sprinkle generously with freshly ground black pepper. I like to keep some fresh, chopped parsley frozen in a plastic container in the freezer so I can just reach for it without having to chop it each time.

1.6 grams of carbohydrate in entire recipe.

Edam Scrambled Eggs

Try Edam Scrambled Eggs with slices of Nova Scotia smoked salmon on the side.

Serves 1

2 eggs
4 tablespoons grated Edam cheese (about 1½ ounces)
1 teaspoon whipped butter
1 teaspoon very light olive oil
Freshly ground black pepper to taste

Break eggs into a bowl and beat thoroughly with a wire whisk. Add grated cheese to eggs. Melt butter and oil in a nonstick skillet, pour in egg mixture, and cook over lowest heat possible until the cheese has melted, stirring frequently. Once the cheese has melted, raise heat to medium and allow eggs to set, raising cooked parts with a spatula to allow uncooked parts to flow to the bottom to cook. When eggs are completely cooked to your taste, remove to a warm plate. Sprinkle with a generous quantity of ground black pepper.

1.5 grams of carbohydrate in entire recipe.

Eggs and Egg Dishes: Thanks to the Chickens

Curried Eggs with Lobster

Lobster, eggs, cream, and curry—yummy! What a lunch!

Makes 1 serving

¼ cup lobster meat, diced
1 teaspoon whipped butter
1 teaspoon very light olive oil
Dash of paprika
¼ to ½ teaspoon curry powder, more or less depending upon the brand of curry powder used
⅛ teaspoon salt
2 eggs
4 teaspoons fat-free half-and-half

Melt the butter and oil in a heavy, nonstick skillet. Add the diced lobster and sauté it for a minute just to heat it. Combine the paprika, curry powder, and salt and add it to the lobster meat. Beat the eggs with the half-and-half only long enough to combine them, then add them to the lobster. Mix them in thoroughly, and continue cooking over low heat just until the eggs begin to set.

3.0 grams of carbohydrate in entire recipe.

Omelets Aplenty

General Directions for Omelet Making

Have a separate pan you use only for omelets. This pan should not be washed once it is seasoned. If anything sticks to the pan, just rub it with a little coarse salt. Otherwise, merely wipe the pan out with a paper towel. I use a nonstick pan that I can put in the dishwasher.

Have the eggs at room temperature. To bring the eggs to

room temperature quickly, immerse them, before cracking, in a bowl of warm water. Wash and dry the eggs and you are ready to make your omelet.

Beat the eggs with either fat-free half-and-half or cold water only long enough to blend them. Do not overbeat or the omelet will be tough. An omelet should contain 2 or 3 eggs only. Do not attempt to use more eggs as it will be too hard to handle.

Heat the omelet pan over high heat until a few drops of water sizzle when sprinkled on it. Lower the flame to medium and put in the butter and oil. Spread the butter around the pan with a fork until it covers the sides and bottom. Add the eggs and make about 8 to 10 circular turns with the fork to raise layers of fluffiness, at the same time shaking the pan back and forth with your hand. Work fast.

When all the liquid has set and the top of the omelet appears glossy, add the filling to the third of the omelet farthest from the handle. Change the position of your hand so that your palm is facing up when you hold the pan and begin rolling the omelet. Raise the handle and gently roll the omelet with the fork. Turn the omelet onto a warm plate by tilting the pan over completely. The entire process should take 1 to 1½ minutes. Serve the omelet immediately while warm.

Caviar Omelet

The epitome of elegance in an omelet.

Makes 1 serving

2 eggs
1 teaspoon fat-free half-and-half
1 tablespoon sour cream, 50 percent reduced fat
1 teaspoon minced chives
1 teaspoon whipped butter
2 teaspoons very light olive oil
2 teaspoons red or black caviar

Beat the eggs lightly with the half-and-half only until blended. Mix together the sour cream and chives and set aside. Make the omelet following general directions on page 177. Turn the omelet onto a warm plate. Top with a dollop of sour cream and chives and place the 2 teaspoons of caviar on top of the sour cream. Serve immediately while warm.

2.6 grams of carbohydrate in entire recipe.

Double Cheese Omelet

Makes 1 serving

2 eggs
1 teaspoon fat-free half-and-half
1 teaspoon grated Parmesan cheese
1 teaspoon butter
2 teaspoons extra-virgin olive oil
1 tablespoon fat-free half-and-half
1 tablespoon grated Gruyère cheese

Break the eggs into a bowl and beat with the teaspoon of half-and-half just until blended. Do not overbeat. Stir in the grated Parmesan cheese. Heat the butter and oil in a nonstick omelet pan and prepare as in General Directions for Omelet Making (page 177). Before folding over the omelet, pour the tablespoon of half-and-half over eggs and sprinkle with grated Gruyère cheese, then turn over onto a plate.

3.2 grams of carbohydrate in entire recipe.

180   THE LOW-CARB GOURMET

Cheese and Herb Omelet

Makes 1 serving

2 eggs
2 teaspoons fat-free half-and-half
2 tablespoons minced parsley
1 tablespoon minced chives
¼ cup grated Gruyère cheese
1 teaspoon whipped butter
2 teaspoons very light olive oil

Beat eggs with half-and-half only enough to blend them. Follow General Directions for Omelet Making (page 177), sprinkling the omelet with parsley, chives, and grated cheese in that order before turning.

2.8 grams of carbohydrate in entire recipe.

NOTE: L'Étoile was a French restaurant in New York that served a lovely buffet brunch on Saturdays and Sundays. When I couldn't decide whether I'd rather have *fines herbes* or cheese in my omelet, the chef suggested I have both. This is the result of his suggestion.

A Favorite Omelet

This title speaks for itself.

Makes 1 serving

2 slices Canadian bacon
2 eggs
1 teaspoon fat-free half-and-half
1 ounce Gruyère cheese (not the processed version)
1 teaspoon chopped chives, fresh, frozen, or freeze-dried
1 teaspoon whipped butter
2 teaspoons light olive oil

Panbroil the Canadian bacon, then cut it in cubes. Break the eggs into a bowl and beat lightly with the half-and-half. Cut the cheese in tiny cubes and add it, Canadian bacon, and chives to the eggs. Mix thoroughly. Heat the butter and oil in a well-seasoned omelet pan or in a nonstick omelet pan and prepare using General Directions for Omelet Making (page 177).

2.0 grams of carbohydrate in entire recipe.

Fines Herbes Omelet

The herb-butter topping makes all the difference.

Makes 1 serving

2 teaspoons whipped butter
4 teaspoons very light olive oil
1 teaspoon fresh chives, minced
1 teaspoon fresh tarragon, minced
1 teaspoon fresh parsley, minced
2 extra-large eggs
1 teaspoon fat-free half-and-half
1 teaspoon fresh chives, minced
1 teaspoon fresh tarragon, minced
1 teaspoon fresh parsley, minced

To make an herb butter, mix together 1 teaspoon each of fresh chives, fresh tarragon, and fresh parsley. Melt half the butter and oil over a low flame and add the seasonings.

Meanwhile beat the eggs with the half-and-half or water only enough to blend them. Add the remaining chives, tarragon, and parsley to the eggs. Make the omelet following General Directions for Omelet Making (page 177). Turn the omelet onto a warm plate and pour the herb butter over it. Serve immediately while warm.

1.4 grams of carbohydrate in entire recipe.

182 THE LOW-CARB GOURMET

Fines Herbes Soufflé Omelet

A puffy version of a Fines Herbes Omelet.

Makes 1 serving

2 extra-large eggs, separated
¼ teaspoon cream of tartar
1 tablespoon fat-free half-and-half
2 tablespoons chopped chives, fresh, frozen, or freeze-dried
2 tablespoons chopped fresh parsley
¼ teaspoon dried tarragon or ½ teaspoon fresh tarragon, if available
1 teaspoon whipped butter
2 teaspoons very light olive oil

Beat egg whites until foamy, add cream of tartar and continue beating until stiff but not dry. Beat the egg yolks lightly with the half-and-half. Add the chives, parsley, and tarragon to the egg yolks. Very gently, fold the beaten egg whites into the egg yolk mixture, being careful not to break down the egg whites. Melt butter and oil in an 8-inch nonstick omelet pan or well-seasoned iron omelet pan. Pour in the eggs. Fry until golden brown on the bottom (yes, you may peek) and set on top. Slide one half of the omelet onto a warm plate, then fold in half. Serve immediately.

2.6 grams of carbohydrate in entire recipe.

Greek Omelet

The Feta cheese gives this omelet a nice Greek touch.

Makes 1 serving

2 eggs
1 teaspoon fat-free half-and-half
1 tablespoon minced parsley

1 teaspoon minced chives
¼ cup crumbled Greek Feta cheese
1 tablespoon extra-virgin olive oil

Beat the eggs with the half-and-half only long enough to blend them. Make the omelet following General Directions for Omelet Making (page 177). Sprinkle the omelet with the herbs, then with the Feta cheese before turning.

2.0 grams of carbohydrate in entire recipe.

Ham Omelet

This omelet was my favorite breakfast at The Gray Gull Inn in Nantucket, Massachusetts.

Makes 1 serving

2 eggs
1 teaspoon fat-free half-and-half
3 tablespoons chopped ham
1 teaspoon whipped butter
2 teaspoons very light olive oil

Beat eggs with half-and-half only enough to blend them. Mix in the chopped ham. Follow General Directions for Omelet Making (page 177).

1.7 grams of carbohydrate in entire recipe.

Ham and Cheese Omelet

Makes 1 serving

1 recipe Ham Omelet (above)
2 tablespoons grated Gruyère cheese

Follow instructions for Ham Omelet, sprinkling the omelet with the grated cheese before turning it.

2.0 grams of carbohydrate in entire recipe.

NOTE: The last time I was in Paris, I ate at an outdoor café that put all of the omelet fillings into the eggs before the eggs went into the pan. I liked it so such that I've been doing it ever since.

Ham-Mushroom Omelet

Makes 1 serving

½ tablespoon olive oil
2 ounces firm white mushrooms—this is about 3 small
 mushrooms or 2 large ones
¼ cup diced ham
1 tablespoon sour cream, 50 percent reduced fat
⅛ teaspoon dried tarragon (You can use ½ teaspoon fresh if
 available)
¼ teaspoon chives, fresh, frozen, or freeze-dried
Dash salt and pepper
2 eggs, at room temperature
1 teaspoon fat-free half-and-half
1 teaspoon whipped butter
2 teaspoons light olive oil

Heat oil in a heavy skillet, add the mushrooms, and sauté them for about two minutes. Add the ham and sauté for 2 to 3 minutes more. The mushrooms should remain rather firm. Lower the flame, mix in the sour cream, tarragon, chives, salt and pepper. Heat only long enough to warm the sour cream.

Beat the eggs with a teaspoon of the half-and-half only enough to blend the eggs. Make omelet following General Directions for Omelet Making (page 177). Before turning, spread the mushroom-ham mixture over the eggs. Turn out onto a warm plate and serve immediately.

5.5 grams of carbohydrate in entire recipe.

Italian Cheese Omelet

A rich, creamy omelet.

Makes 1 serving

2 eggs
2 teaspoons water
1 tablespoon extra-virgin olive oil
2 ounces ricotta—a scant ¼ cup
1 ounce finely chopped or grated mixed Italian cheeses

Have all ingredients at room temperature. Beat the eggs with the water only long enough to combine them. Follow General Directions for Omelet Making (page 177) filling the omelet with the ricotta and then with the mixed cheeses before turning it.

4.2 grams of carbohydrate in entire recipe.

NOTE: You may include any Italian cheeses you have on hand but try to include a little mozzarella and grated Parmesan. I combine any or all of the following—mozzarella, Parmesan, Bel Paese, Fontina, Teleggio, and Provolone.

THE LOW-CARB GOURMET

Mushroom, Herbs, and Cheese Omelet

Madame Romaine de Lyon is a restaurant in New York that serves authentic French omelets with hundreds of different flavorings. This is one of the ones I have eaten there.

Makes 1 serving

3 medium-size mushrooms
1 tablespoon very light olive oil
1 tablespoon chopped chives, fresh or frozen
2 eggs
2 teaspoons fat-free half-and-half
½ cup grated Swiss Emmenthal cheese
1 teaspoon whipped butter
2 teaspoons very light olive oil

Sauté the mushrooms in 1 tablespoon oil. Remove from heat, add the chives, and set aside. Beat the eggs with the half-and-half only long enough to blend them. Make the omelet following General Directions for Omelet Making (page 177), spreading the eggs with the mushrooms and then the cheese before turning it.

6.6 grams of carbohydrate in entire recipe.

Mushroom Soufflé Omelet

Makes 1 serving

¼ pound firm white mushrooms, thinly sliced
1 tablespoon extra-virgin olive oil
½ teaspoon lemon juice
¼ teaspoon salt
Generous dash of freshly ground black pepper
2 extra-large eggs, at room temperature, separated
¼ teaspoon cream of tartar
1 tablespoon fat-free half-and-half

Eggs and Egg Dishes: Thanks to the Chickens

Another dash of freshly ground black pepper
1 teaspoon whipped butter
2 teaspoons light olive oil

Sauté the mushrooms in 1 tablespoon oil with the lemon juice, salt, and pepper.

Beat egg whites until foamy, add cream of tartar, and continue beating until stiff but not dry. Beat egg yolks lightly with the half-and-half and a little freshly ground pepper. Very gently fold the beaten whites into the yolk mixture, being careful not to break down the whites.

Melt butter and oil in an 8-inch nonstick pan or well-seasoned omelet pan. Pour in the eggs.

Fry until golden brown on the bottom (yes, you may peek) and set on top. Spread with the sautéed mushrooms, reserving about 1 tablespoon of mushrooms as a garnish. Slide half of the omelet onto the center of a warm plate, then fold the remaining half over the top. Garnish with the reserved mushrooms. Serve immediately.

7.6 grams of carbohydrate in entire recipe.

Cheese, Tomato, and Herb Omelet

Serve this omelet unfolded like an Italian frittata.

Makes 1 serving

2 teaspoons very light olive oil
1 teaspoon whipped butter
½ medium-size tomato, sliced thinly
2 eggs
1 teaspoon fat-free half-and-half
2 teaspoons water
Salt and freshly ground pepper to taste
1 teaspoon chives, minced
1 teaspoon parsley, minced
2 ounces Gruyère cheese, grated

Place the butter and oil in a 6- to 7-inch nonstick skillet and heat to sizzling. Arrange the tomato slices in the butter in a single layer. Beat the eggs with the half-and-half, water, salt and pepper only long enough to combine them and add them to the pan, raising the tomato slices to allow the eggs to run to the bottom of the pan. Sprinkle the top with the chives and parsley, then with the grated Gruyère cheese. Continue to cook the eggs over a low flame only long enough for the cheese to melt.

6.8 grams of carbohydrate in entire recipe.

Soufflés

Cheese Soufflé

The first soufflé I ever made was a miserable failure, but I only failed once, so don't be discouraged! You'll soon be making high, light, and puffy ones.

Makes 4 servings

1 tablespoon whipped butter
1 tablespoon very light olive oil
2 tablespoons full-fat soy flour
½ cup fat-free half-and-half
½ cup cold water
½ teaspoon salt
Dash of white pepper
¾ cup (about 3 ounces) grated, sharp Cheddar cheese
Dash of nutmeg
Dash of cayenne pepper
2 egg yolks
6 whole eggs, at room temperature, separated
¾ teaspoon cream of tartar

Preheat oven to 400° F. Butter a 6-cup soufflé dish. Make a waxed paper or foil collar for it, and set it aside.

Melt butter and oil in a heavy saucepan over low heat. With a wire whisk, stir in the soy flour. Cook for a few minutes until thoroughly blended. Combine half-and-half and water and add slowly to the butter-flour mixture, stirring constantly with the whisk. Add the salt and pepper and heat to scalding. Then add the cheese, nutmeg, and cayenne. When the cheese has melted, beat in the 2 egg yolks, 1 at a time. Heat a few more minutes, but do not allow mixture to boil. Remove from the heat. Separate the remaining 6 eggs and beat in the yolks, 1 at a time. Beat egg whites until foamy, add cream of tartar, and continue beating until stiff but not dry. Fold about a fourth of the egg whites into the cheese sauce thoroughly, then very gently fold in the remainder, being careful not to break the whites down. Turn soufflé batter into the prepared dish and bake 25 to 30 minutes. Remove from the oven and serve immediately.

19.7 grams of carbohydrate in entire recipe; if serving 4, each serving contains 4.9 grams of carbohydrate.

Gourmet Soufflé

Swiss Gruyère and Parmesan are my favorite combination of cheeses for a soufflé.

Makes 4 to 5 servings

Follow directions for Cheese Soufflé (page 188), adding 1 cup of grated Gruyère cheese (approximately ¼ pound), and ¼ cup grated Parmesan cheese in place of the Cheddar cheese. Bake the soufflé at 425° F. for 25 minutes.

19.7 grams of carbohydrate in entire recipe; if serving 4, each serving contains 4.9 grams of carbohydrate.

Münster-Caraway Soufflé

Makes 4 servings

1 tablespoon whipped butter
1 tablespoon light olive oil
2 tablespoons full-fat soy flour
½ cup fat-free half-and-half
½ cup cold water
Dash of cayenne pepper
½ teaspoon salt, or to taste
Dash of white pepper
1 cup diced Münster cheese (¼ pound)
½ teaspoon caraway seeds
2 egg yolks
4 whole eggs
1 extra egg white
½ teaspoon cream of tartar

Follow directions for Cheese Soufflé (page 188) substituting Münster cheese for Cheddar cheese. Add the caraway seeds to the cheese sauce. Bake in a 1½-quart soufflé dish at 375° F. for 30 to 35 minutes.

20.3 grams of carbohydrate in entire recipe; if serving 4, each serving contains 5.0 grams of carbohydrate.

VIII.

Vegetables and Salads: Gifts from the Earth

Baked Artichoke Hearts 193
Green Beans Amandine 194
My Mother's Stuffed Cabbage 194
Cauliflower with Cheese 196
Fried Cauliflower 196
Braised Sliced Celery 197
Celery Gruyère 198
My Mother's Stuffed Eggplant Roll 198
Broiled Eggplant Slices 200
Braised Endive 200
Sautéed Escarole 201
Mock Pasta 202
Creamed Mushrooms with Cheese 203
My Mother's Stuffed Green Peppers 203
Creamed Spinach 205
Sautéed Spinach 206
Grilled Tomatoes with Cheese 206
French Fries 207
My Mother's Stuffed Zucchini 208
Zucchini with Cheese 210
Salade Niçoise 210
Fresh Salmon Salad Niçoise 211
Bacon, Spinach, and Mushroom Salad 212
Chef's Salad 213
Coleslaw 214
Sweet-and-Sour Cucumber Salad 214
Green Bean Salad 215
Potato-like Salad 216
French Potato-like Salad 217

Vegetables and Salads: Gifts from the Earth

I could have given many more recipes for fancy ways to prepare vegetables; however, I feel that it's a crime to doctor them up too much. The trick to making vegetables delicious is to avoid overcooking them. Do as the Chinese do and use color as a guide to judging when the vegetables are cooked. Green vegetables should remain bright green; when they become dull, it means they are overcooked. Use a steamer, pressure cooker, or heavy saucepan placed over high heat with very little water, and, above all, keep the vegetables crisp. Picture crisp asparagus, broccoli, green beans, zucchini, or cauliflower with melted butter—heaven on earth!

Baked Artichoke Hearts

Makes 3 servings

1 box frozen artichoke hearts
Salt
1 tablespoon extra-virgin olive oil
2 teaspoons whipped butter, melted
¼ cup grated Parmesan cheese

Preheat oven to 350° F. Cook artichokes in salted water for 5 minutes. Mix together the oil and melted butter. Drain artichoke hearts thoroughly and place in a shallow 7-inch baking dish. Pour the oil-butter mixture over them and mix in thoroughly. Bake for 5 minutes at 350° F., then raise the oven

194   THE LOW-CARB GOURMET

temperature to 450° F., top artichokes with Parmesan cheese, and bake for 10 to 12 minutes.

14.3 grams of carbohydrate in entire recipe; if serving 3, each serving contains 4.8 grams of carbohydrate.

Green Beans Amandine

A delicate, delicious method for preparing green beans.

Makes 5 servings

1 pound very tiny green beans
2 quarts water
1 tablespoon salt
2 tablespoons very light olive oil
2 teaspoons whipped butter
3 tablespoons slivered almonds, toasted
Additional salt and freshly ground pepper to taste

Trim the ends from the beans. Bring water to a boil, add salt and beans, then return to boil and cook beans, uncovered, for 8 to 10 minutes. Beans should be crisp-tender. Test 1 by eating it. Set the color by running beans under cold water. Dry with paper towels. Warm oil and butter in a skillet, add the beans, and toss in the mixture. Add the toasted almonds. Serve hot.

34.0 grams of carbohydrate in entire recipe; if serving 5, each serving contains 6.8 grams of carbohydrate.

My Mother's Stuffed Cabbage

Makes 12 cabbage bundles

12 large cabbage leaves
1 pound very lean ground beef

Vegetables and Salads: Gifts from the Earth

1 egg
1 tablespoon minced onion
¼ teaspoon salt, or to taste
Generous sprinkling of freshly ground black pepper
Artificial sweetener equal to ⅛ teaspoon sugar
⅔ cup tomato sauce
¼ teaspoon salt
Dash of freshly ground black pepper
2 tablespoons fresh lemon juice
2 cups cold water
Artificial sweetener equal to 3 tablespoons sugar
Brown sugar artificial sweetener equal to 1 tablespoon brown sugar

Buy a large, very loose head of cabbage, as the leaves will be easier to separate. Soften cabbage leaves in boiling water for 5 minutes, then remove, and drain thoroughly.

Mix together the ground beef, egg, minced onion, ¼ teaspoon of salt, black pepper, and artificial sweetener equal to ⅛ teaspoon sugar. Divide the meat into 12 equal parts. Place 1 part on 1 cabbage leaf, tuck in the sides, and carefully roll it up. Repeat this procedure until all 12 leaves are rolled. Carefully tie each cabbage bundle with heavy-weight, white sewing thread (6 or 8 cord), to hold together during cooking.

In a heavy saucepan, combine the tomato sauce, ¼ teaspoon salt, dash of pepper, lemon juice, cold water, and both artificial sweeteners. Bring this mixture to a boil and carefully place cabbage bundles in it. Cover the pot, lower the flame, and simmer 1 hour. Taste sauce and correct seasoning. The sauce should be both sweet and sour. Serve hot with sauce spooned over the bundles. Stuffed cabbage can be served either as an appetizer or as a main course.

35.0 grams of carbohydrate in entire recipe; makes 12 cabbage bundles, each one containing 2.9 grams of carbohydrate. These figures are based upon the cabbage being served with the sauce.

Cauliflower with Cheese

Makes 6 servings

1 large cauliflower (about 3 pounds before trimming)
Salt
1 tablespoon whipped butter, melted
1 tablespoon very light olive oil
¼ pound grated sharp white Cheddar cheese
Freshly ground black pepper to taste

Preheat oven to 400° F. Cook the cauliflower whole in salted water to cover 20 to 25 minutes until crisp-tender. Drain thoroughly. Place the cauliflower in a round snugly fitting baking dish. A soufflé dish is nice for this. Dot the cauliflower with whipped butter and oil mixture and grated cheese. Bake until the cheese melts and browns slightly. Sprinkle with black pepper and serve immediately.

30.5 grams of carbohydrate in entire recipe; if serving 6, each serving contains 5.1 grams of carbohydrate.

Fried Cauliflower

A dressed-up version of cauliflower.

Makes 8 servings

1 large cauliflower (3 pounds before trimming), cooked crisp-tender
2 tablespoons Seasoned Soy Flour (page 29)
2 extra-large eggs
2 tablespoons oil
2 teaspoons butter

Separate the cooked cauliflower into flowerets. Dredge flowerets lightly in the Seasoned Soy Flour. Beat the eggs, then dip the flowerets into the eggs. Heat the oil and butter together in a heavy skillet, add the cauliflower, and fry until golden brown on all sides. Serve immediately.

34.5 grams of carbohydrate in entire recipe; if serving 8, each serving contains 4.3 grams of carbohydrate.

Braised Sliced Celery

Makes 3 servings

2 tablespoons light olive oil
1 tablespoon whipped butter
1 pound celery stalks sliced at a diagonal (about 5 cups)
3 tablespoons chicken broth
½ teaspoon salt
Generous dash of freshly ground black pepper

Melt butter and oil in a heavy skillet over medium heat. Add sliced celery and mix thoroughly for 2 to 3 minutes until celery is completely coated with butter-oil mixture. Add chicken broth, salt, and pepper, cover the pan, and cook for 10 to 12 minutes until celery is crisp-tender and the pan juices have thickened. Serve hot.

13.6 grams of carbohydrate in entire recipe; if serving 3, each serving contains 4.5 grams of carbohydrate.

Celery Gruyère

Cooked celery blends well with cheese.

Makes 3 servings

Place 1 recipe Braised Sliced Celery (page 197) in a baking dish. Pour the pan juices over the celery. Sprinkle with ¼ cup grated Swiss Gruyère cheese and place under the broiler until the cheese melts and browns.

14.1 grams of carbohydrate in entire recipe; if serving 3, each serving contains 4.7 grams of carbohydrate.

My Mother's Stuffed Eggplant Roll

This is a Mideast specialty, a bit complicated to make, but definitely worth the trouble.

Makes 12 rolls

1 3-pound elongated eggplant
Salt
3 pounds very lean ground beef
3 tablespoons minced onion
1 teaspoon salt
Freshly ground black pepper to taste
Artificial sweetener equal to ⅜ teaspoon sugar
6 extra-large eggs
5 tablespoons Seasoned Soy Flour (page 29)
4 tablespoons oil

Sauce

2 cups tomato sauce
¼ cup lemon juice
Artificial sweetener equal to ¼ cup sugar
Brown sugar artificial sweetener equal to 1 tablespoon
  brown sugar

Peel the eggplant, then slice it lengthwise into ¼-inch slices making sure to remove the seeds. Sprinkle each slice lightly on both sides with salt and place in a deep bowl. The salt will soften the eggplant and make it give off its water. Allow to sit at least 1 hour. Meanwhile, mix together stuffing ingredients—beef, onion, salt, pepper, artificial sweetener, and 3 eggs—and set aside.

Squeeze any remaining water from the eggplant by pressing the slices with paper towels. Reserve the 12 broadest center slices of eggplant. Cut up the remaining eggplant slices and place them over the center parts of the eggplant. Divide the meat mixture into 12 equal parts and place 1 part on each slice of eggplant. Roll up slices and tie each with 6 or 8 cord white thread.

Beat remaining 3 eggs. Dredge each eggplant roll in Seasoned Soy Flour (page 29), then dip in beaten egg. Heat 2 tablespoons of the oil in each of 2 large skillets and fry rolls until golden brown on all sides.

In a shallow 3½-quart casserole, heat together the tomato sauce, lemon juice, and remaining artificial sweeteners. Add eggplant rolls to the sauce, cover pan, lower flame to simmer, and cook 1 hour. To serve, spoon sauce over the eggplant rolls and serve hot.

113.9 grams of carbohydrate in entire recipe; makes 12 eggplant rolls, each containing 9.5 grams of carbohydrate.

Broiled Eggplant Slices

Try this recipe on an outdoor grill if you have a backyard or a terrace.

Makes 4 servings

1 1-pound eggplant
6 tablespoons olive oil
2 tablespoons mild wine vinegar
1 clove garlic, crushed
Generous sprinkling of freshly ground black pepper
Salt

Slice the eggplant into ½-inch slices. Combine olive oil, vinegar, garlic, and pepper. Place eggplant slices on a sheet of aluminum foil or on a broiling pan, brush with half the oil and vinegar mixture, and broil until golden brown. Turn the slices, brush with the remaining oil and vinegar, and broil until the other side is golden brown. Remove from the heat, sprinkle with salt, and serve hot.

22.6 grams of carbohydrate in entire recipe; if serving 4, each serving contains 5.7 grams of carbohydrate.

Braised Endive

Endive is as delicious served hot as a vegetable as it is when served cold in a salad.

Makes 6 servings

2 pounds endive
3 tablespoons extra-virgin olive oil

1 tablespoon whipped butter
½ cup chicken stock

Wash endive, then dry in paper towels. Melt the butter and oil in a large, heavy skillet. Add endive to the pan and roll in the melted butter and oil until all pieces are completely coated. Add chicken stock, cover pan, and cook over low heat 40 to 45 minutes or until liquid has evaporated and endive is golden brown. Turn the endive to brown all sides. Serve hot.

26.5 grams of carbohydrate in entire recipe; if serving 6, each serving contains 4.4 grams of carbohydrate.

Sautéed Escarole

Makes 8 servings

2 pounds escarole
2 tablespoons olive oil
2 cloves garlic, minced
½ teaspoon oregano
Salt and freshly ground pepper to taste

Wash escarole in deep water in a clean sink. Repeat 2 or 3 times more. Dry with paper towels or in a salad spinner. Heat a nonstick pan and add the oil and garlic to the pan. Add the escarole and sauté until tender or about 10 minutes. Mix in the oregano, salt and pepper to taste and cook for another 1 or 2 minutes. Serve hot.

33.6 grams of carbohydrate in entire recipe; if serving 8, each serving contains 4.2 grams of carbohydrate.

Mock Pasta

Makes 3 servings

1½ quarts water
2 teaspoons salt
1½ teaspoons oregano
1 teaspoon basil
¼ teaspoon onion powder
2 dashes garlic powder
¼ teaspoon freshly ground pepper
1 can Chinese bean sprouts
2–3 tablespoons extra-virgin olive oil
1–1½ cloves fresh garlic, crushed
¼ cup chopped fresh parsley
Chopped fresh basil (optional)
¼ cup grated Parmesan cheese
Salt and freshly ground pepper to taste

Combine first 7 ingredients and bring to a boil. Add bean sprouts and return to a boil. Lower flame and simmer 20 minutes. Drain in a colander. Return bean sprouts to the pan and dry for 1 minute over high heat. Over high flame, toss with oil. Add garlic and remove from heat. Add parsley, fresh basil, and cheese and toss. Season with salt and freshly ground pepper to taste. Serve with additional grated Parmesan cheese.

12.2 grams of carbohydrate in entire recipe; if serving 3, each serving contains 4.1 grams of carbohydrate.

Creamed Mushrooms with Cheese

Try serving these mushrooms with a simple grilled steak and a tossed green salad.

Makes 4 servings

2 tablespoons light olive oil
1 tablespoon whipped butter, unsalted
1 pound firm, white fresh mushrooms, thinly sliced
2 tablespoons dry sherry
¼ cup sour cream, 50 percent reduced fat
2 tablespoons freshly grated Parmesan cheese
Salt and freshly ground pepper to taste
Additional Parmesan cheese, if desired

Melt butter in a skillet. Add oil. Add sliced mushrooms and sauté 2 minutes. Add sherry and cook 1 minute more. Mix together sour cream, grated cheese, salt and pepper and add to mushrooms. Cook over a low flame until sour cream has warmed thoroughly (do not boil). Add additional grated cheese, if desired. Serve warm.

25.6 grams of carbohydrate in entire recipe; if serving 4, each serving contains 6.4 grams of carbohydrate.

My Mother's Stuffed Green Peppers

Makes 8 large peppers

8 large green peppers

Stuffing

3 pounds very lean ground beef
3 tablespoons minced onion
¾ teaspoon salt, or to taste
3 eggs
Generous sprinkling of freshly ground black pepper
Artificial sweetener equal to ⅜ teaspoon of sugar

Sauce

1⅓ cups tomato sauce
¾ teaspoon salt
Generous sprinkling of freshly ground black pepper
¼ cup fresh lemon juice
2 cups cold water
Artificial sweetener equal to ¼ cup sugar
Brown sugar artificial sweetener equal to 2 tablespoons
   brown sugar

Cut a ½-inch piece across stem end of peppers and carefully remove all fibers and seeds. Wash and dry the peppers and set aside.

Mix together the ground beef, minced onion, salt, eggs, freshly ground black pepper, and artificial sweetener equal to ⅜ teaspoon sugar. Divide meat into 8 equal parts and stuff pepper cavities with it, pressing the meat down to the very bottom.

In a heavy saucepan, combine tomato sauce, ¾ teaspoon salt, freshly ground black pepper, lemon juice, cold water, and remaining artificial sweetener. Bring this mixture to a boil, then place the stuffed peppers in it. Cover pot, lower flame, and simmer 1 hour. Taste the sauce and correct seasoning.

Remove the stuffed peppers to a warm platter. Raise flame under the sauce, and boil to reduce and thicken. Spoon thickened sauce over the stuffed peppers and serve hot. You may serve the peppers whole or cut them in half lengthwise.

68.8 grams of carbohydrate in entire recipe; makes 8 peppers, each pepper containing 8.6 grams of carbohydrate.

NOTE: These figures are based upon the peppers being served with the sauce. Stuffed peppers can be served either as an appetizer or as a main course, depending upon the size of the portions. One whole pepper makes a full main course.

Creamed Spinach

Guaranteed to make people who hate spinach learn to love it.

Makes 4 servings

2 packages frozen chopped spinach
1 teaspoon salt
3 tablespoons cold water
½ cup fat-free half-and-half
2 egg yolks
Generous dash of freshly ground nutmeg
Generous dash of freshly ground black pepper
Additional salt, if necessary

Cook the spinach with the salt and water, covered, over high heat for approximately 4 minutes or until just defrosted. (Do not follow the directions on the package.) If there is any liquid left in pan, remove the cover and continue cooking 1 or 2 minutes more until liquid evaporates. Mix together the half-and-half and egg yolks and add to spinach. Cook over low heat, stirring constantly, until spinach combines well with the cream mixture and thickens (do not boil). Season to taste with the nutmeg, pepper, and more salt if necessary.

29.6 grams of carbohydrate in entire recipe; if serving 4, each serving contains 7.4 grams of carbohydrate.

Sautéed Spinach

The Italian method for preparing spinach.

Makes 6 servings

2 pounds fresh spinach
2 tablespoons olive oil
2 cloves of garlic, minced
½ teaspoon salt
Generous dash of freshly ground black pepper

Follow directions for Sautéed Escarole (page 201), cutting the cooking time down to 5 to 6 minutes.

28.8 grams of carbohydrate in entire recipe; if serving 6, each serving contains 4.8 grams of carbohydrate.

Grilled Tomatoes with Cheese

The inspiration for this recipe came from Elizabeth David, England's gift to the world of food.

Serves 4

½ pound Swiss Gruyère cheese
3 tablespoons dry white wine or vermouth
Generous dash freshly ground black pepper
Dash of cayenne
Dash of Dijon-style mustard
1 small clove garlic, put through a press
4 medium-size tomatoes
Salt

Preheat oven to 350° F. Cube the cheese and place it in a heavy saucepan over very low heat. Mix in the wine, black pepper, cayenne, mustard, and garlic. Heat until cheese melts and all ingredients are well blended, stirring frequently.

While the cheese is melting, cut off the tops from 4 medium-size tomatoes. Scoop out the pulp and seeds. Sprinkle the tomato shells with salt, turn them upside down and allow them to drain. Fill each tomato shell with about 3 tablespoons of the melted cheese mixture. Place the tomatoes in individual ramekins if possible, as it is difficult to pick them up later. Bake for 10 minutes, then remove them to the broiler and broil for a few minutes until the cheese mixture browns lightly. Serve immediately.

20.8 grams of carbohydrate in entire recipe; makes 4 tomatoes, each containing 5.2 grams of carbohydrate.

French Fries

White turnips make a great substitute for potatoes in French Potato-like Salad and in this recipe. Try to obtain small white turnips. They have a much milder flavor than the larger ones.

Makes 4 servings

6 small white turnips, approximately 1 pound
Extra-virgin olive oil
Herbs de Provence (see page 16)
Salt and freshly ground pepper to taste

Preheat oven to 450° F. Wash and dry the turnips; if the skins are clean and free of bruising, you will not have to peel them. Slice turnips lengthwise in both directions into ½-inch sticks. Place in a single layer on a nonstick cookie sheet or on a cookie sheet covered with Release aluminum foil. Sprinkle lightly with extra-virgin olive oil, then with herbs de

Provence and freshly ground pepper. Bake for approximately 15 to 17 minutes or until light golden brown, then turn them. Add a little more herbs de Provence and continue baking for another 15 to 17 minutes until all sides are golden brown.

Remove to paper towels to drain off any excess oil. Sprinkle very lightly with salt and serve while hot. You can dip these into ketchup containing 1 gram of carbohydrate per tablespoon if you really want to, but taste them first. You may find that you don't need it.

25.7 grams of carbohydrate in entire recipe; if serving 4, each serving contains 6.4 grams of carbohydrate.

My Mother's Stuffed Zucchini

My mother spent four years in the Middle East before she was married. This is one of the specialties she learned to make while she was there. It's my favorite of all her stuffed vegetable recipes!

Makes 16 pieces

4 1-pound zucchini (each 9–10 inches long)

Stuffing

1 pound very lean ground beef
¼ teaspoon salt
Generous dash of freshly ground black pepper
1 tablespoon minced onion
Artificial sweetener equal to ⅛ teaspoon sugar
1 egg

Sauce

⅔ cup tomato sauce
¼ teaspoon salt, or to taste

Vegetables and Salads: Gifts from the Earth

Dash of freshly ground black pepper
2 tablespoons fresh lemon juice
1 cup cold water
Artificial sweetener equal to 3 tablespoons sugar
Brown sugar artificial sweetener equal to 1 tablespoon brown sugar

Trim the ends from the zucchini, then wash and dry. Do not peel. Cut each zucchini in two 4½- to 5-inch pieces. Scoop out each piece with an apple corer, discarding seeds and reserving flesh. Shells should be ¼ inch thick at sides and bottom.

For stuffing, mix together the ground beef, salt, black pepper, egg, minced onion, and artificial sweetener equal to ⅛ teaspoon of sugar. Divide the meat into 8 equal parts and stuff zucchini cavities with it, pressing the meat down to the very bottom.

Make sauce in a heavy saucepan, combining tomato sauce, ¼ teaspoon salt, pepper, lemon juice, cold water, and artificial sweeteners. Bring this mixture to a boil, add reserved zucchini flesh, then lay the stuffed zucchini on top. Cover pot, lower flame, and simmer 1 hour.

Taste the sauce (which may need salt) and correct seasoning. Remove stuffed zucchini to a warm platter and cut each one in half crosswise, to make 16 pieces. Raise flame under the sauce, and boil to reduce and thicken. Spoon thickened sauce over the stuffed zucchini and serve hot. The zucchini scoopings will have become part of the sauce.

72.7 grams of carbohydrate in entire recipe; makes 16 pieces, each piece containing 4.5 grams of carbohydrate.

NOTE: These figures are based upon the zucchini being served with the sauce. Stuffed zucchini can be served either as an appetizer or as a main course, depending upon the size of the portions.

Zucchini with Cheese

Makes 4 servings

1½ pounds 5–6-inch zucchini
Salt
1 tablespoon extra-virgin olive oil
3 tablespoons grated Parmesan cheese
Generous dash of freshly ground pepper

Trim the ends from the zucchini, but do not peel. Cook whole in salted water to cover, 6 to 8 minutes, then drain. Slice zucchini into 1-inch rounds. Warm oil in a skillet, add zucchini, and toss lightly. Remove to a warm serving dish and stir in Parmesan cheese. Sprinkle with the freshly ground pepper. Serve hot.

24.0 grams of carbohydrate in entire recipe; if serving 4, each serving contains 6.0 grams of carbohydrate.

Salade Niçoise

My version of a delicious French main-dish salad. This salad was the hit of our beach house when served with Beach House Mustard Dressing (page 260).

Makes 4 servings

10 large leaves romaine lettuce
3 6½-ounce cans tuna fish, flaked
12 anchovy fillets, halved
12 black olives
½ cup cooked green beans
3 hard-cooked eggs, quartered
2 small tomatoes, quartered
8 marinated artichoke hearts

Vegetables and Salads: Gifts from the Earth

Arrange the lettuce leaves on a large platter. Mix together all remaining ingredients and arrange on the lettuce. Serve with Vinaigrette Dressing (page 260) or Beach House Mustard Dressing.

24.3 grams of carbohydrate in entire recipe; if serving 4, each serving contains 6.1 grams of carbohydrate.

NOTE: This recipe can also be used in smaller portions as an appetizer as is frequently done in France.

Fresh Salmon Salad Niçoise

This recipe was inspired by Eli's Fresh Salmon Salad in a Tomato Wrap. Eli's is a gourmet shop and restaurant in New York that also distributes their wonderful Sour Dough Bread and Rolls to other gourmet shops. I've added the raspberry vinegar, as it's great with salmon, and I left out the wrap and made it as a salad plate. I also made the little red potatoes optional, since they're very high on the Glycemic Index.

Makes 4 servings

1½ pounds poached fresh salmon (or leftover grilled salmon)
1 red pepper, cut lengthwise into ⅛-inch slices
1 yellow or orange pepper, cut lengthwise into ⅛-inch slices
1 large stalk celery, cut diagonally into ¼-inch slices
4 plum tomatoes, each cut into 6 pieces
20 small green beans, blanched, cut into quarters
4 scallions, each cut into ¼-inch pieces
4 cups torn romaine lettuce or mesclun
8 black olives, pitted and halved
24 capers
4 tiny red potatoes, cooked and quartered (optional, if your diet allows these)

212   THE LOW-CARB GOURMET

Raspberry Vinaigrette Dressing

8 tablespoons (½ cup) extra-virgin olive oil
4 tablespoons (¼ cup) raspberry vinegar
1 tablespoon Dijon-style mustard
Salt and freshly ground pepper to taste

Cut the salmon into pieces about ¾ inch in diameter. Combine with the peppers, celery, tomatoes, green beans, scallions, lettuce or mesclun, olives, capers, and—if you are using them—the red potatoes. Beat together the ingredients for the dressing and add it to the salad ingredients. Lightly toss the salad ingredients and the dressing together.

57.2 grams of carbohydrate in entire recipe; if serving 4, each serving contains 14.3 grams of carbohydrate. Add 4.0 grams of carbohydrate to entire recipe if using the potatoes, and divide that number by four if serving four people.

Bacon, Spinach, and Mushroom Salad

Try this as a main-dish luncheon salad.

Makes 8 servings

1 pound bacon
1 pound fresh spinach
1 pound small, firm, white mushrooms
¾ cup olive oil
¼ cup mild wine vinegar
2 tablespoons chopped fresh parsley
½ teaspoon Dijon-style mustard
½ teaspoon salt
Generous sprinkling of freshly ground black pepper

Broil bacon until crisp and drain on paper towels. Trim heavy stems from the spinach and wash thoroughly. Dry thoroughly in paper towels or in a salad spinner. Wipe mushrooms with a damp cloth or paper towel and slice. Mix spinach leaves and mushrooms together and crumble broiled bacon over all. Place the oil, vinegar, parsley, mustard, salt, and pepper in a blender and blend a few seconds at high speed. Toss the salad with this dressing.

41.6 grams of carbohydrate in entire recipe; if serving 8, each serving contains 5.2 grams of carbohydrate.

Chef's Salad

A perennial favorite for lunch or dinner.

Makes 2 servings

¼ pound imported Swiss Emmenthal cheese
¼ pound ham
¼ pound cooked white meat of chicken
6–8 lettuce leaves
2 hard-cooked eggs, halved
4 green pepper rings
16 thin slices cucumber
1 small tomato cut into wedges
2 scallions

Slice the cheese, ham, and chicken into Julienne strips about 2 to 3 inches long. Arrange lettuce on 2 plates, making a bed for the remaining ingredients. Divide all the ingredients in half. Arrange little piles of cheese, ham, and chicken on each plate, then decorate with the eggs and vegetables. Each plate should contain some of each of the ingredients. Serve with Vinaigrette Dressing (page 260), Roquefort Dressing (page 261), or mayonnaise.

24.4 grams of carbohydrate in entire recipe; if serving 2, each serving contains 12.2 grams of carbohydrate.

214   THE LOW-CARB GOURMET

Coleslaw

Makes 4 servings

1 pound cabbage
¼ cup white vinegar
1 tablespoon white wine vinegar
2 tablespoons fresh lemon juice
½ cup sugarless mayonnaise
Artificial sweetener equal to 1 tablespoon sugar
2 tablespoons grated green pepper
2 tablespoons grated sweet red pepper
Salt and freshly ground pepper to taste

Shred cabbage very fine and place in a large bowl. Add the vinegars, lemon juice, mayonnaise, and artificial sweetener and toss lightly. Mix in the 2 kinds of pepper and add salt and freshly ground black pepper to taste. Place in an attractive serving dish, cover with plastic wrap, and refrigerate until serving time. Coleslaw goes particularly well with fish.

30.4 grams of carbohydrate in entire recipe; if serving 4, each serving contains 7.6 grams of carbohydrate.

Sweet-and-Sour Cucumber Salad

A refreshing change from the usual tossed salad. Try these cucumbers when serving a rich main course.

Serves 4

2 long, narrow cucumbers
½ cup white vinegar
½ cup cold water
½ teaspoon salt

Dash of black pepper
Artificial sweetener equal to 1 tablespoon sugar

Peel cucumbers and slice as thin as possible. If you get very narrow cucumbers, this can easily be done with a vegetable peeler. Combine vinegar, cold water, salt, pepper, and artificial sweetener and pour this mixture over sliced cucumbers. Marinate overnight in the refrigerator. These cucumbers are particularly good when serving any main dish made with sour cream.

19.2 grams of carbohydrate in entire recipe; if serving 4, each serving contains 4.8 grams of carbohydrate.

Green Bean Salad

A favorite vegetable becomes a salad.

Makes 5 servings

1 pound tiny green beans
2 quarts water
1 tablespoon salt
6 tablespoons olive oil
2 tablespoons mild wine vinegar
3 tablespoons chopped chives, fresh or frozen
Salt and freshly ground pepper to taste

Trim the ends from the beans. Bring water to a boil, add salt and beans, return to boil, and cook, uncovered, 8 to 10 minutes. Beans should be crisp-tender. Test 1 by eating it. Set the color by running the beans under cold water, then dry. Mix together oil, vinegar, and chives with salt and pepper to taste. Pour dressing over the beans and refrigerate for at least 2 hours.

29.9 grams of carbohydrate in entire recipe; if serving 5, each serving contains 6.0 grams of carbohydrate.

Potato-like Salad

I've fooled more people with this recipe. A number of people agreed that this was the best-tasting potato salad they had ever eaten, without even knowing there wasn't a potato in it!

Serves 8

2 pounds small white turnips, or larger ones, halved
2 teaspoons salt
2 tablespoons beef broth—may be made with bouillon cube
2 tablespoons dry white wine
6 tablespoons sugarless mayonnaise
2 tablespoons sour cream, 50 percent reduced fat
4 teaspoons Dijon-style mustard
2 dashes ground celery seed
1 hard-cooked egg
2 tablespoons finely minced onion
2 tablespoons finely minced celery
4 teaspoons finely minced green pepper
4 tablespoons minced parsley
Salt and freshly ground pepper to taste

Peel the turnips and place in water to cover. Add salt, bring to a boil, lower flame, and cook 20 to 25 minutes until turnips test done with a fork. Remove turnips from the water and dry on paper towels, then cut in small cubes.

Combine the broth and wine and toss turnips with this mixture while still warm. Combine mayonnaise, sour cream, mustard, and celery seed. When the turnips have stood in the wine mixture 10 minutes, add sour cream–mayonnaise, and toss lightly. Dice the hard-cooked egg and add along with the onion, celery, green pepper, and parsley. Lightly toss again. Add salt and pepper to taste. Chill briefly and serve.

58.9 grams of carbohydrate in entire recipe; if serving 8, each serving contains 7.4 grams of carbohydrate.

NOTE: Potato-like Salad or even real potato salad should never be served icy cold for best flavor. If you are making this in advance, take it out of the refrigerator at least an hour before serving time. See how many people will really believe that they're eating real potato salad if you don't tell them!

French Potato-like Salad

For those who like their potato salad European-style—without mayonnaise.

Makes 8 servings

2 pounds small white turnips, or large ones, halved
2 teaspoons salt
2 tablespoons beef broth—may be made with bouillon cube
2 tablespoons dry white wine
2 tablespoons white wine vinegar
¼ teaspoon salt
1 teaspoon Dijon-style mustard
6 tablespoons olive oil
2 tablespoons minced scallions
¼ cup minced parsley
Dash black pepper

Peel the turnips and place in water to cover. Add salt, bring to a boil, lower flame, and cook 20 to 25 minutes until the turnips test done with a fork. Remove turnips from the water and dry on paper towels, then cut in thin slices.

Combine the broth and wine and toss the sliced turnips with this mixture while still warm so they will absorb the flavor. Combine vinegar, salt, and mustard and beat to dissolve the salt. Beat in the oil, a little at a time, until all 6 tablespoons are used. Add minced scallions and parsley to the dressing with a dash or two of freshly ground black pepper. Pour the dressing over the turnips and toss lightly to avoid breaking the slices.

55.0 grams of carbohydrate in entire recipe; if serving 8, each serving contains 6.9 grams of carbohydrate.

IX.

A Visit to Asia

Chinese Egg Drop Soup 222
Chinese Salad Dressing or Shrimp Dip 223
Chinese Chicken Salad 223
Chinese Beef and Vegetable Salad 224
Chinese Stuffed Mushrooms 225
Chinese Stuffed Peppers 226
Chinese Stuffed Cucumbers 227
Chinese Stuffed Cabbage 228
Dietetic Chinese Duck Sauce 230
Chinese Roast Pork 230
Chinese Pork and Cucumbers 231
Chinese Barbecued Spareribs 232
Chinese Beef and Broccoli 233
Chinese Beef and Asparagus 234
Chinese Pepper Steak 235
Beef with Chinese Vegetables 236
Chinese Chicken and Cauliflower 237
Chinese Chicken and Peppers 238
Chinese Shrimp Egg Foo Yong 238
Chinese Barbecued Shrimp and Livers 240
Chinese Shrimp with Cucumbers 240
Chinese Shrimp with Peppers and Mushrooms 241
Chinese Shrimp and Broccoli 242
Japanese Grilled Beef (Beef Teriyaki) 242
Japanese Grilled Salmon (Salmon Teriyaki) 243
Sukiyaki 244
Chicken Sukiyaki 245
Vegetable Sukiyaki 247

A Visit to Asia

Asian food has always been popular in this country. Chinese food, when properly prepared, can be low in carbohydrates. Most American Chinese restaurants use far too much cornstarch to thicken their sauces. This extra cornstarch not only adds no flavor and thickens the gravy to a gluelike consistency, it adds unwanted grams of carbohydrates. In China, the food is not thickened to the degree that it is in our restaurants. I have cut the amounts of cornstarch customarily used without sacrificing flavor and, more important, kept the carbohydrate count low.

In this chapter, I have often purposely omitted mentioning the number of servings for each recipe. Since Chinese food is usually served family-style, with a number of dishes placed on the table to be shared, just add up the carbohydrate and calorie values for each of the dishes you are serving and divide those numbers by the number of people you are serving.

In many of the recipes, I have used the expression *stir-fry* to describe the cooking method for that particular dish. *Stir-fry* is actually another word for *sauté*. In effect, the ingredients are sautéed quickly over high heat, with the food being stirred constantly by holding a pancake turner in one hand and a ladle or basting spoon in the other. The motion is similar to tossing a salad.

Asian food is a special delight to me and has been one of my favorite things since I was a child. In the section "Some Useful Ingredients for Low-Carbohydrate Cooking," page 17 at the front of this book, I have included some tips for special Asian ingredients, which will be helpful to you when you are trying these recipes.

Chinese Egg Drop Soup

Do you know anybody who doesn't like Chinese Egg Drop Soup? When we were teenagers, my mother would let my sister and me go to the Chinese restaurant by ourselves every Saturday night. How grown-up we felt!

Serves 8

2 eggs
2 teaspoons water
2 scallions
6 cups chicken stock, fresh, canned, or made with a cube
1 teaspoon dry sherry
1 tablespoon Chinese light or Japanese soy sauce,
    50 percent reduced salt
Salt to taste—use less with a packaged broth mix
Artificial sweetener equal to ½ teaspoon sugar

Beat eggs and stir in water. Set aside. Mince scallions and set aside. Bring chicken stock to a boil. Reduce heat to medium and stir in sherry, soy sauce, and salt. Pour eggs in slowly, a little at a time, so that soup continues to boil at all times. Keep stirring constantly, till eggs separate into shreds. A wire whisk is good for this. Remove from heat and stir in artificial sweetener. Garnish with minced scallions.

Any of the following ingredients may be added if desired: soaked, dried black mushrooms, bamboo shoots, lean pork, sesame oil, black pepper, shredded chicken, or 2 more teaspoons dry sherry.

5.0 grams of carbohydrate in entire recipe; if serving 8, each serving contains 0.6 grams of carbohydrate.

Chinese Salad Dressing or Shrimp Dip

Even if this mixture sounds odd to you, try it. You'll never be sorry.

Makes 1 cup plus 2 tablespoons dressing

6 tablespoons soy sauce, 50 percent reduced salt
6 tablespoons Chinese rice vinegar, or mild cider or wine vinegar
6 tablespoons Chinese sesame oil
2 teaspoons dry mustard

Combine all ingredients and mix well.

This delightful dressing can be used as a dip for cold shrimp to be served as an appetizer or for Chinese cold salads. If you have never tried a Chinese cold salad, try this on Chinese Chicken Salad (below) and you'll be converted for life.

12.9 grams of carbohydrate in entire recipe; makes 18 tablespoons, each tablespoon containing 0.7 grams of carbohydrate.

Chinese Chicken Salad

The Chinese certainly can cook, but who would have dreamed of a Chinese chicken salad?

Makes 8 appetizer servings or 4 luncheon-dish servings

2 whole chicken breasts, cooked
1 large cucumber or 2 small; or 2 stalks celery
½ recipe Chinese Salad Dressing (above)

Using fingers, shred the 2 chicken breasts (the shredding gives texture). Cut up the cucumbers or celery—whichever one you are using—and place on a pretty serving plate. Place shredded chicken on top of cucumbers. Bring the dressing to the table separately and toss the salad with the dressing just before serving.

13.1 grams of carbohydrate in entire recipe if cucumbers are used (10.5 grams if using celery); if serving 8, each serving would contain 1.6 grams (1.3 with celery).

Chinese Beef and Vegetable Salad

Another version of a Chinese cold salad.

Makes 4 appetizer servings

2 teaspoons Chinese dark or Japanese soy sauce, 50 percent reduced salt
2 teaspoons dry sherry
½ teaspoon cornstarch
½ pound beef, sliced very thinly in small strips
2 tablespoons oil
¼ pound cabbage, washed, shredded, and sprinkled with ½ teaspoon salt
¼ pound fresh tomatoes, sliced, then shredded
1 tablespoon soy sauce, 50 percent reduced salt
1 teaspoon ginger juice
1½ teaspoons Chinese sesame oil

Combine 2 teaspoons soy sauce, sherry, and cornstarch and marinate beef in this mixture 5 minutes. Heat a wok or large frying pan for 30 seconds, add the oil, and heat another 30 seconds over high heat. Add the beef and stir-fry (sauté) until color changes. Remove from pan and cool.

Squeeze any excess water from the cabbage, and arrange on a serving platter in this way: an outside ring of cabbage, the center filled with shredded tomato, and the beef on top of the tomato, leaving a thin ring of tomato showing outside of the meat. Mix the soy sauce, ginger juice, and sesame oil together and place in a small bowl to be taken to the table separately. Toss the salad with the dressing before serving. This salad should be served cold and can be made in advance.

16.2 grams of carbohydrate in entire recipe; if serving 4 as an appetizer, each serving contains 4.1 grams of carbohydrate.

Chinese Stuffed Mushrooms

If you've never tasted the dried Chinese mushrooms, you're in for a treat. They're marvelously meaty and tasty.

Makes 4 appetizer servings

12 large, dried Chinese mushrooms
½ pound very lean ground pork
4 teaspoons Chinese dark or Japanese soy sauce, 50 percent reduced salt
4 teaspoons very dry sherry
¼ teaspoon salt
Dash of black pepper
1 teaspoon Chinese sesame oil

Soak the mushrooms in warm water for 15 to 30 minutes. Combine ground pork with soy sauce, sherry, salt, pepper, and Chinese sesame oil and mix thoroughly. After mushrooms are softened, remove stems. Divide pork into 12 equal parts. Stuff the mushroom caps with the pork mixture, mounding the tops. Arrange the stuffed mushrooms on a heat-proof plate. Place on a steaming rack and steam for 15 minutes. Serve the stuffed mushrooms with Chinese mustard and/or soy sauce.

14.3 grams of carbohydrate in entire recipe; makes 12 mushrooms, each mushroom containing 1.2 grams of carbohydrate; if serving 4, each serving contains 3.6 grams of carbohydrate.

NOTE: To improvise a steamer if you do not have one, place a cake rack in a pot. Place boiling water under the rack, and then place the dish containing the food to be steamed on top of the cake rack. Cover the pot, keeping the flame about medium to avoid burning the pot, and steam the food.

Chinese Stuffed Peppers

Makes 4 appetizer servings

½ pound very lean ground pork or beef
1 extra-large egg
2 teaspoons Chinese dark or Japanese soy sauce, 50 percent reduced salt
2 teaspoons dry sherry
1 large scallion, minced
½ teaspoon salt
1 slice fresh ginger (1-inch diameter), minced
2 large green peppers, halved
2 tablespoons peanut oil
½ cup water
2 teaspoons Chinese dark or Japanese soy sauce, 50 percent reduced salt
Granulated artificial sweetener equal to 1 teaspoon sugar

To make the stuffing, mix together meat, egg, soy sauce, sherry, scallion, salt, and ginger. Divide the meat mixture into 4 equal parts and fill each green pepper half, stuffing the meat well into the pepper cavities. Heat a wok or large frying pan 30 seconds, add the oil, heat over high heat for another 30 seconds. Add the peppers, meat side down, and fry 2 minutes, then turn meat-side up and fry 1 minute. Add water and dark soy sauce and cook over low heat 10 minutes. Remove peppers to a serving platter, raise heat if necessary, and cook down the sauce a little. Remove from heat and stir in artificial sweetener. Pour sauce over peppers and serve hot.

10.5 grams of carbohydrate in entire recipe; if serving 4 as an appetizer, each serving contains 2.6 grams of carbohydrate. The carbohydrate count remains the same whether you use pork or beef.

Chinese Stuffed Cucumbers

Another version of a stuffed vegetable.

Makes 4 appetizer servings

1 very large or 2 small cucumbers
1 recipe stuffing for Chinese Stuffed Peppers (page 226)
2 tablespoons peanut oil
¼ cup chicken stock
2 teaspoons dry sherry
1 teaspoon Chinese dark or Japanese soy sauce, 50 percent reduced salt
¼ teaspoon salt
Granulated artificial sweetener equal to ½ teaspoon sugar

Peel the cucumbers and cut to make 4 lengthwise sections. Scoop seeds out carefully. Prepare stuffing mix and fill hollowed cucumbers. Heat a wok or frying pan 30 seconds, add the oil, and heat over a high flame another 30 seconds. Add the cucumbers meat-side down. Fry 2 minutes, turning so that sides are cooked evenly. Add sauce ingredients: stock, sherry, soy sauce, and salt. Cook, covered, for 20 minutes.

Remove cucumbers to a serving platter and cook sauce a few more minutes to reduce and/or thicken it. Remove from heat and stir in artificial sweetener Pour the sauce over cucumbers and serve hot.

11.8 grams of carbohydrate in entire recipe; if serving 4 as an appetizer, each serving contains 3.0 grams of carbohydrate. The carbohydrate count remains the same whether you use pork or beef.

Chinese Stuffed Cabbage

Every nationality has its stuffed cabbage and here's the Chinese version.

Makes 8 cabbage rolls

8 leaves Chinese celery cabbage

Stuffing

½ pound very lean beef, ground
¼ cup finely chopped onion
½ teaspoon salt
2 teaspoons Chinese dark or Japanese soy sauce, 50 percent reduced salt
2 teaspoons dry sherry

Sauce

⅓ cup juice from the cabbage after steaming
1 teaspoon Chinese dark or Japanese soy sauce, 50 percent reduced salt
1 teaspoon Chinese rice vinegar or mild wine or cider vinegar
½ teaspoon cornstarch, mixed with 1 teaspoon cold water
Artificial sweetener equal to 2 teaspoons sugar

Boil the celery cabbage leaves for about 5 minutes, rinse under cold water to stop further cooking, and drain thoroughly. Cut the leaves in 4- to 5-inch sections and reserve the excess trimmings.

Combine ground meat with onion, salt, soy sauce, and sherry and mix thoroughly. Divide the meat into 8 equal portions, and place 1 in the center of each leaf section. Fold the sides of the leaves over to make neat rolls. Cut the excess trimmings of celery cabbage into ½-inch slices and line a heat-proof bowl with them. Place the cabbage rolls on top. Steam the rolls for 15 minutes, then remove to a serving platter. See Chinese Stuffed Mushrooms (page 225) for directions if you need to improvise a steamer.

Prepare sauce in a small pan, combining ⅓ cup of the juice left after steaming cabbage and add dark soy sauce, rice vinegar, and cornstarch and bring to a boil, stirring constantly. Boil for a few minutes just to thicken sauce a little. Remove from the heat and stir in the artificial sweetener. Pour the sauce over the stuffed cabbage and serve.

14.9 grams of carbohydrate in entire recipe; makes 8 cabbage rolls, each cabbage roll containing 1.9 grams of carbohydrate.

NOTE: If Chinese celery cabbage is not available, regular round cabbage leaves may be substituted.

Dietetic Chinese Duck Sauce

A must for Chinese Roast Pork or Chinese Barbecued Spareribs.

Makes 1 cup

5 ounces sugar-free, artificially sweetened apricot jam
1 ounce artificially sweetened strawberry jam
5 tablespoons Chinese rice vinegar (or substitute a mild cider vinegar or a mild wine vinegar)
1 tablespoon minced fresh gingerroot
3–4 cloves fresh garlic, crushed
½ teaspoon Chinese dark or Japanese soy sauce, 50 percent reduced salt
⅛ teaspoon hot red pepper flakes
1 teaspoon chili powder

Combine all ingredients, mix thoroughly, and refrigerate for a few hours or overnight to help develop the flavor. Use as a dip for Chinese food. This sauce keeps well in the refrigerator.

13.9 grams of carbohydrate in entire recipe; makes 1 cup of sauce, each tablespoon containing 0.9 grams of carbohydrate.

Chinese Roast Pork

Makes 8 appetizer servings, 4 main course servings

2 pounds boneless pork tenderloin
2 tablespoons dry sherry
2 tablespoons dark soy sauce, 50 percent reduced salt
Brown sugar substitute equal to 2 tablespoons regular brown sugar

1 teaspoon salt
½ teaspoon Chinese Five-Spice Powder*
1 large or 2 small cloves of garlic, minced
2 slices fresh ginger (1-inch diameter), slivered
1 large scallion, cut in 1-inch pieces
Few drops of red food coloring (optional, but nice)

Cut pork into 2 strips lengthwise. Combine remaining ingredients in a shallow bowl or pie plate and mix thoroughly. Place meat in marinade, cover with plastic wrap or foil, refrigerate, and let meat marinate for at least 3 hours or overnight. Turn meat in the marinade once in a while.

Remove pork strips from marinade. Roast under a hot broiler 1 hour, turning frequently. Baste frequently with the remaining marinade. May be eaten hot or cold with Chinese mustard or Dietetic Chinese Duck Sauce (page 230).

8.2 grams of carbohydrate in entire recipe; if serving 8 as an appetizer, each serving contains 1.0 grams of carbohydrate. If serving 4 as a main course, each serving contains 2.0 grams of carbohydrate.

Chinese Pork and Cucumbers

½ pound lean pork
Marinade of 2 teaspoons soy sauce, ½ teaspoon cornstarch, and 1 teaspoon dry sherry
2 cups sliced large cucumbers, or whole small pickling cucumbers
2 tablespoons peanut oil
1 tablespoon soy sauce, 50 percent reduced salt
Artificial sweetener equal to ½ teaspoon sugar
Dash of salt

*If you cannot obtain Chinese Five-Spice Powder, you can make it by combining equal parts of powdered cinnamon, powdered cloves, aniseed, and thyme—or substitute ½ teaspoon plain cinnamon.

Cut the pork into very thin slices or tiny cubes. Place in marinade for 5 minutes. Wash cucumbers; if large, peel, seed, and slice at a diagonal; if small pickling variety, dry and use whole without peeling. Heat a wok or large frying pan, add oil, wait about 30 seconds, then add pork. Stir-fry the pork over high heat until the color changes. Add the remaining ingredients and continue to stir-fry for another 1 to 2 minutes. Serve hot.

10.9 grams of carbohydrate in entire recipe.

Chinese Barbecued Spareribs

An old favorite of my childhood Chinese restaurant days.

Makes 6 appetizer servings

1 2-pound rack of spareribs
2 tablespoons Chinese dark or Japanese soy sauce, 50 percent reduced salt
2 tablespoons very dry sherry
2 tablespoons sugar-free, artificially sweetened, orange marmalade
2 tablespoons sugar-free, artificially sweetened, strawberry jam
1 teaspoon salt
4 slices fresh ginger (1-inch diameter), minced
4 large cloves of garlic, minced
2 scallions, cut in 1-inch pieces
Few drops red food coloring (optional, but nice)

If possible, try to obtain small spareribs. Do not separate them; leave them as a rack, but have the butcher crack the bones. Combine remaining ingredients, mix well, and marinate the spareribs in this mixture. For convenience, use a large plastic bag and turn the entire bag over to turn the spareribs in the marinade. Place a plate underneath the plastic bag in case any of the liquid leaks. Marinate ribs at least 4 hours or overnight, turning occasionally.

Preheat oven to 350° F. Separate ribs, place in a shallow roasting pan (I like to use a disposable pan) and bake 1 hour and 15 minutes, basting frequently with any remaining marinade. The spareribs should now be browned; if not, turn oven up to 475° F. for 5 or 10 minutes. Serve with Chinese mustard or Dietetic Chinese Duck Sauce (page 230).

11.0 grams of carbohydrate in entire recipe; if serving 6 as an appetizer, each serving contains 1.8 grams of carbohydrate.

Chinese Beef and Broccoli

Chinese meals are both quick and delicious. This recipe even uses convenient frozen broccoli.

¾ pound flank steak
2 tablespoons soy sauce, 50 percent reduced salt
1 tablespoon dry sherry
½ teaspoon cornstarch
1 package frozen broccoli, defrosted
1 clove garlic, minced
1 thin slice fresh ginger (1-inch diameter), finely minced
2 tablespoons peanut oil
Salt to taste

Slice the steak against the grain into very thin slices. Combine the soy sauce, sherry, and cornstarch and pour this mixture over the steak. Marinate the meat for 15 minutes.

While the meat is marinating, slice the broccoli at a diagonal and mince garlic and ginger. Heat a wok or large frying pan for 30 seconds, add oil, wait about 20 seconds, and add minced garlic and gingerroot. Fry over high heat, stirring constantly for about 20 seconds more, then add the beef. Stir-fry, stirring constantly, for about 1 minute. Add broccoli and stir-fry for another 4 to 6 minutes, until the broccoli is cooked but still crisp and still dark green. Serve hot.

18.4 grams of carbohydrate in entire recipe.

Chinese Beef and Asparagus

If you thought that the only way to eat asparagus was with hollandaise, this may surprise you.

¾ pound flank steak
1½ tablespoons soy sauce, 50 percent reduced salt
1 teaspoon dry sherry
Granulated artificial sweetener equal to ½ teaspoon sugar
½ teaspoon cornstarch
2 tablespoons peanut oil
1 cup water
½ pound fresh asparagus (see NOTE)
1 tablespoon shredded scallion
¼ teaspoon salt, or to taste

Slice the steak against the grain in very thin slices. (This is easily done by slicing the meat when it is slightly frozen.) Combine the soy sauce, sherry, artificial sweetener, and cornstarch and pour this mixture over beef. Marinate the steak 15 minutes.

While the meat is marinating, trim off the tough lower end of asparagus stalks and slice asparagus at a diagonal. Boil water, drop asparagus into it, and when water returns to boil, cook 2 minutes. Drain the asparagus.

Heat a wok or large frying pan for 30 seconds, add oil, count to 30, add scallion and beef, and stir-fry over high heat about 1 minute. Add asparagus and salt and continue to stir-fry for 2 more minutes.

10.7 grams of carbohydrate in entire recipe.

NOTE: You may substitute one package of frozen asparagus if fresh is not available. Then do not boil, merely defrost.

Chinese Pepper Steak

¾ pound lean beef
Marinade of 2 teaspoons soy sauce, artificial sweetener
   equal to ½ teaspoon sugar, 1 teaspoon dry sherry, and
   ½ teaspoon cornstarch
1½ green peppers
½ red pepper
1 slice fresh ginger (1-inch diameter)
2 tablespoons peanut oil
1 tablespoon soy sauce (50 percent reduced salt) mixed
   with 1 teaspoon dry sherry

Slice the beef into thin strips and place in marinade for 15 minutes.

While the meat is marinating, slice peppers thinly and mince the ginger. Mix together the seasonings and set aside.

Heat a wok or large frying pan for 30 seconds, add 1 tablespoon of the oil, continue heating for another 30 seconds over high heat. Add the peppers and stir-fry 2 minutes. Remove peppers to a warm plate.

Add the remaining tablespoon of oil to the wok, heat 30 seconds more, add the ginger, and heat until golden brown. Add beef and stir-fry until the color of beef changes. Return peppers to the pan, add soy-sherry seasoning and continue to stir-fry for another minute or 2 until all ingredients are thoroughly mixed. Serve hot.

10.9 grams of carbohydrate in entire recipe.

Beef with Chinese Vegetables

½ pound lean beef
Marinade of 1 teaspoon soy sauce (50 percent reduced salt), 1 teaspoon dry sherry, and ½ teaspoon cornstarch
1 clove garlic, minced
1 slice fresh ginger, minced
4 dried Chinese mushrooms, soaked 30 minutes in warm water
6–8 snow peas
3 water chestnuts, each sliced in 3 slices
¼ cup bamboo shoots, sliced

Seasonings Mixture

2 teaspoons soy sauce, 50 percent reduced salt
2 teaspoons dry sherry
Artificial sweetener equal to ½ teaspoon sugar
2 tablespoons peanut oil

Slice the beef into thin strips and place in marinade 15 minutes.

While the meat is marinating, mince the garlic and ginger, slice the mushrooms into thin strips, remove the string from the snow peas, and slice the water chestnuts. Mix together the seasonings. Heat a wok or large frying pan for 30 seconds, add 1 tablespoon of oil, and continue heating for another 30 seconds over high heat. Add the vegetables and stir-fry for 2 minutes. Remove them to a warm plate.

Add the remaining tablespoon of oil, heat 30 seconds more, add the meat, and stir-fry until meat changes color. Return the vegetables to the pan, add seasoning mixture, and blend thoroughly. Cook for 1 or 2 minutes more until thoroughly combined. Serve hot.

15.8 grams of carbohydrate in entire recipe.

Chinese Chicken and Cauliflower

Definitely one of the fastest yet most delicious ways of preparing chicken that I've ever tasted.

1 skinless, boneless chicken breast (about 8 ounces)
2 tablespoons soy sauce, 50 percent reduced salt
1 tablespoon dry sherry
Granulated artificial sweetener equal to 1 teaspoon sugar
½ teaspoon cornstarch
3 tablespoons minced cooked ham
1 tablespoon Chinese parsley (regular parsley may be substituted)
1 package frozen cauliflower, defrosted
2 tablespoons peanut oil
2 tablespoons water
Salt to taste

Cut the raw chicken breast in thin slices. Combine the soy sauce, sherry, artificial sweetener, and cornstarch and pour over chicken. Marinate the chicken in this mixture 10 minutes.

While chicken is marinating, chop ham and parsley. Pour boiling water over cauliflower, leave 1 minute, drain, and set aside.

Heat a wok or large frying pan for 30 seconds, add the oil, count to 30, and add chicken slices. Stir-fry chicken over high heat for about 2 minutes. Add cauliflower and continue stir-frying another 2 minutes. Add water and salt to taste and cover tightly. Cook 5 minutes. Remove to a serving dish, and sprinkle parsley and ham on top.

13.1 grams of carbohydrate in entire recipe.

Chinese Chicken and Peppers

1 skinless, boneless chicken breast (about 8 ounces)
Marinade of 1 teaspoon dry sherry and ½ teaspoon cornstarch
1½ green peppers
½ red pepper
1 tablespoon dry sherry
½ teaspoon salt
Granulated artificial sweetener equal to ½ teaspoon sugar
3 tablespoons peanut oil

Slice the chicken breast into thin slices. Marinate the chicken in sherry and cornstarch for 5 minutes. Halve the peppers, seed, and slice into very thin slices. Combine 1 tablespoon of sherry, ½ teaspoon salt, and the artificial sweetener and set aside.

Heat a wok or large frying pan for 30 seconds, add 1 tablespoon of the oil, wait 30 seconds, add peppers, and stir-fry for 2 minutes. Remove peppers to a plate. Add remaining 2 tablespoons of oil, and stir-fry chicken until it turns white. Return the peppers to pan, add the seasonings mixed earlier and continue to stir-fry until all ingredients are well mixed (about 1 minute). Serve immediately.

7.9 grams of carbohydrate in entire recipe.

Chinese Shrimp Egg Foo Yong

Makes 8 pancakes

Sauce

¾ cup chicken broth
1 tablespoon soy sauce, 50 percent reduced salt
½ teaspoon cornstarch
Additional salt if desired

Pancakes

½ pound shrimp, shelled and deveined
¼ pound fresh mushrooms
3 extra-large eggs
1 tablespoon peanut oil
½ cup bean sprouts
¼ teaspoon salt
1 teaspoon dry sherry
Artificial sweetener equal to ¼ teaspoon sugar
1½ tablespoons additional peanut oil

To make the sauce, bring the chicken broth to a boil. Add soy sauce and cornstarch. Boil 1 to 2 minutes until sauce turns clear and thickens slightly. Keep warm over very low heat while you make pancakes.

Dice the shrimp and mushrooms into ¼-inch pieces. Beat the eggs in a bowl. Heat a wok or frying pan for 30 seconds, add 1 tablespoon of the oil, and continue heating for another 30 seconds. Add shrimp and stir-fry until pink. Add the sautéed shrimp to the eggs, then add the mushrooms and bean sprouts to the eggs along with salt, sherry, and artificial sweetener.

Brush the bottom of the same wok or of a 5- or 6-inch frying pan with 1 teaspoon oil, reduce flame to low, and pour in approximately ¼ cup of the egg-shrimp batter. Allow it to cook for 1 minute without touching it. When lightly browned (you may peek), turn it, and cook another minute or so until that side is lightly browned, too. Remove to a warm plate and cover with aluminum foil to keep warm. Repeat until all 8 pancakes are made, brushing the pan with ½ teaspoon oil before making each new pancake. Serve hot with the sauce spooned over the pancakes.

14.4 grams of carbohydrate in entire recipe; makes 8 pancakes, each pancake contains 1.8 grams of carbohydrate.

Chinese Barbecued Shrimp and Livers

Makes 4 servings

1 pound large shrimp, shelled and deveined
5 strips bacon
½ pound chicken livers
½ clove garlic
2 slices fresh ginger (1-inch diameter)
½ cup soy sauce, 50 percent reduced salt
¼ cup dry sherry
½ teaspoon salt
Dash of pepper
Granulated artificial sweetener equal to 1½ tablespoons sugar

Butterfly the shrimp. Cut each bacon strip into 4 pieces. Cut each chicken liver in half. Arrange the flattened shrimp in a dish. Place a piece of chicken liver on each shrimp, then top each piece of liver with a piece of the bacon. Mince the garlic and gingerroot. Combine soy sauce, sherry, salt, pepper, and artificial sweetener with the ginger and garlic. Pour over the shrimp and let stand for 20 to 30 minutes. Thread skewers with the shrimp, chicken livers, and bacon in layers. Broil or barbecue the skewers, turning frequently until the shrimp turn pink.

23.4 grams of carbohydrate in entire recipe; if serving 4, each serving contains 5.9 grams of carbohydrate.

Chinese Shrimp with Cucumbers

1 pound uncooked shrimp, shelled and deveined
1 teaspoon dry sherry
2 teaspoons salt

Granulated artificial sweetener equal to 1 teaspoon sugar
½ teaspoon cornstarch
2 medium cucumbers or 3 small pickling cucumbers
2 tablespoons peanut oil
1 tablespoon additional dry sherry

Wash and dry shrimp. Mix together the sherry, salt, artificial sweetener, and cornstarch and marinate the shrimp in this mixture 15 minutes. While the shrimp are marinating, prepare cucumbers: if small pickling variety, just wash and dry; if larger ones, peel, seed, and quarter lengthwise. Slice cucumbers in 1-inch slices.

Heat a wok or large frying pan for 30 seconds, add 1 tablespoon of oil, wait 30 seconds more, add cucumbers, and stir-fry until slightly transparent (3 to 5 minutes). Remove cucumbers to a plate. Add remaining oil and stir-fry the shrimp until pink. Return cucumbers to the pan, add additional sherry, and continue to stir-fry for another 2 minutes. Serve hot.

20.3 grams of carbohydrate in entire recipe.

Chinese Shrimp with Peppers and Mushrooms

½ pound shrimp, shelled and deveined
½ teaspoon ginger juice (page 21)
½ teaspoon cornstarch
½ cup green peppers, cut in ½-inch squares
½ cup fresh mushrooms, cut in ½-inch squares

Seasonings Mixture

2 teaspoons dry sherry
½ teaspoon salt
Granulated artificial sweetener equal to 1 teaspoon sugar
2 tablespoons peanut oil

Marinate shrimp 5 minutes in the ginger juice and cornstarch. Meanwhile, cut the peppers and mushrooms. Combine the seasonings and set aside.

Heat a wok over high heat for 30 seconds, then add oil, wait another 30 seconds for the oil to become very hot, and stir-fry the shrimp until bright pink. Add the peppers and mushrooms and stir-fry for another 2 minutes. Add the seasonings mixed earlier and continue to stir-fry for another 2 or 3 minutes.

9.9 grams of carbohydrate in entire recipe.

Chinese Shrimp and Broccoli

Follow recipe for Chinese Shrimp with Peppers and Mushrooms (page 241), substituting half a package of frozen broccoli, defrosted in advance, for the peppers and mushrooms. Slice the broccoli stems in diagonal slices and separate the flowerets into mouth-size pieces.

12.7 grams of carbohydrate in entire recipe.

Japanese Grilled Beef (Beef Teriyaki)

In Japan, they hand-tend their cattle for their famous Kobe beef to make this dish.

Makes 3 servings

⅓ cup Japanese soy sauce, 50 percent reduced salt
1 tablespoon sake or dry sherry
Artificial sweetener equal to 4½ tablespoons sugar
1 small clove of garlic, minced
1½ pounds lean beef sirloin or tenderloin, sliced ½-inch thick
2 teaspoons peanut oil
3 green peppers, each cut vertically in 3 pieces

Mix together the soy sauce, sake, artificial sweetener, and garlic. Marinate the beef in this mixture 15 minutes. Brush a heavy griddle or frying pan with the oil. Grill the beef and peppers until done to taste. Cook peppers alone first if you like your meat rare. If you have an outdoor grill, try this on it. A grill pan with ridges or an electric grill would also be good.

17.1 grams of carbohydrate in entire recipe; if serving 3, each serving contains 5.7 grams of carbohydrate.

Japanese Grilled Salmon (Salmon Teriyaki)

Another version of teriyaki.

Makes 3 servings

Follow the directions for Japanese Grilled Beef (page 242), substituting fresh salmon fillet slices for the beef. You can omit the peppers and substitute a different vegetable. Just count the carbohydrates in the vegetable you choose.

7.3 grams of carbohydrate in entire recipe; if serving 3, each serving contains 2.4 grams of carbohydrate.

Sukiyaki

Makes 5 to 6 servings

1 cup beef stock
½ cup sake or dry sherry
5 tablespoons Japanese soy sauce, 50 percent reduced salt
Artificial sweetener equal to ½ cup sugar
2 pounds lean beef sirloin or tenderloin, sliced paper thin
¾ pound mushrooms, thinly sliced
8 scallions, cut in 2-inch lengths
1 pound Chinese celery cabbage, sliced in ½-inch rounds
4 cakes bean curd (tofu), cut into 1-inch cubes
1 tablespoon peanut oil

Combine in a small bowl or pitcher the beef stock, sake, soy sauce, and artificial sweetener and set aside. This is the sauce that the other ingredients will be cooked in.

Slice the beef into paper-thin slices. (This is more easily done if the meat is partially frozen.) Have 2 large trays ready and arrange half the meat on each tray. Divide in the same way the sliced mushrooms, scallions, celery cabbage, and bean curd cubes. Form a decorative design with the different ingredients as you arrange them; Japanese people give a great deal of attention to making their food look beautiful.

Sukiyaki is customarily cooked at the table with a little of the ingredients added at a time. Have ready an electric skillet or a small electric 1-burner stove that can be brought to the table with a wide heavy casserole. Oil the pan thoroughly with the peanut oil. Cover the pan bottom with a few beef slices and brown them on both sides. Push the meat to 1 side, then add some of each of the vegetables and some cooking sauce. Continue cooking over low heat. Serve the food and eat it while you cook more. Just add more beef, vegetables, bean curd, and sauce as the food is removed. Serve green tea in small Japanese cups with the Sukiyaki.

55.5 grams of carbohydrate in entire recipe; if serving 6, each serving contains 9.3 grams of carbohydrate.

Chicken Sukiyaki

I've come to prefer Chicken Sukiyaki to Beef Sukiyaki. I personally find the beef too well done in this dish for my taste. However, the Japanese restaurant we go to makes a wonderful Chicken Sukiyaki and a wonderful Vegetable Sukiyaki. They are among my favorite dishes there. On a cold winter's night, when you are not feeling quite up to par, this is so soothing. It's the equivalent of really good Jewish chicken soup and just as therapeutic. On nights when I'm feeling fine I eat it just because I enjoy it so much.

Makes 5 to 6 servings

1 cup beef stock
½ cup sake or dry sherry (a medium-dry Amontillado is fine for this)
5 tablespoons Japanese soy sauce, 50 percent reduced salt
Artificial sweetener equal to ½ cup sugar
2 pounds boneless chicken, sliced very thin
½ pound fresh white mushrooms, thinly sliced
¼ pound Asian mushrooms, fresh, canned, or dried (reconstitute the dried ones in warm water), sliced if large, left whole if small
8 scallions, cut into 2-inch lengths
1 pound celery cabbage
4 carrots, sliced into thick slices
15 small broccoli flowers
4 cakes bean curd (tofu), cut into 1-inch cubes
1 tablespoon peanut oil

Combine in a small bowl or pitcher the beef stock, sake or sherry, soy sauce, and artificial sweetener and set aside. This is the sauce that the other ingredients will be cooked in.

Slice the chicken into thin strips. (This is more easily done if the chicken is partially frozen.) Have 2 large trays ready and arrange ½ the chicken on each tray. Divide in the same way the sliced mushrooms, scallions, celery cabbage, carrots, broccoli, and bean curd cubes. Form a decorative design with the different ingredients as you arrange them; Japanese cooks give a great deal of attention to making their food look beautiful.

Sukiyaki is customarily cooked at the table with a little of the ingredients added at a time. Have ready an electric skillet or a small electric 1- or 2-burner stove that can be brought to the table with a wide, heavy casserole. Oil the pan thoroughly with the peanut oil. Cover the pan bottom with a few chicken slices and brown them on both sides. Push the meat to one side, then add some of each of the vegetables and some cooking sauce, along with some of the bean curd. Continue cooking over low heat. Serve the food and eat it while you cook more. Just add more chicken, vegetables, bean curd, and sauce as the food is removed. Serve green tea or jasmine tea in small Japanese cups with the Chicken Sukiyaki.

70.8 grams of carbohydrate in entire recipe; if serving 6, each serving contains 11.8 grams of carbohydrate.

NOTE: If you are really not feeling well, the best thing you can do if you have a good Japanese restaurant near you that is not wildly expensive, would be to call them and have them deliver some Chicken Sukiyaki to you while you get some rest and pamper yourself or let your family pamper you.

Vegetable Sukiyaki

Sometimes I enjoy this as much as I enjoy Chicken Sukiyaki, particularly if I've had chicken a day or two earlier. I like variety; I don't like to eat the same thing day after day, even if it's prepared differently.

Makes 5 to 6 servings

Follow the directions for Chicken Sukiyaki (page 245), omitting the chicken and adding 4 extra cakes of bean curd. Another thing you can do if you don't want the extra bean curd would be to have a seafood or meat appetizer for the extra protein.

84.0 grams of carbohydrate in entire recipe using the extra bean curd; if serving 6, each serving contains 14.0 grams of carbohydrate.

X.

Sauces, Dressings, and Toppings: A Few Little Things

White Sauce 251
Spiced Cranberry Sauce 252
Apricot Sauce for Duck or Chicken 252
Blackberry Sauce for Duck or Chicken 253
Mint Jelly 254
Mint Sauce 255
Curry Sauce for Seafood 256
Dilled Shrimp Sauce 256
Garlic and Parsley Sauce for Shrimp 257
Mayonnaise Verte 258
Creamy Mustard Sauce 259
Cheese Sauce 259
Vinaigrette Dressing 260
Beach House Mustard Dressing 260
Roquefort Dressing 261
Cinnamon-Sugar Topping 262
Pesto Sauce 262
Nutted Cheese Spread 263

Sauces, Dressings, and Toppings: A Few Little Things

Here are a variety of sauces, salad dressings, and toppings for sweet things. These are what dress up your cooking and can make the difference between the ordinary and the extraordinary.

White Sauce

Use this white sauce whenever a recipe calls for regular white sauce.

Makes 1 cup

1 tablespoon butter
1 tablespoon very light olive oil
2 tablespoons full-fat soy flour
½ cup fat-free half-and-half
½ cup cold water
Salt to taste
Dash of white pepper
2 egg yolks

Melt butter in a heavy saucepan over low heat. Add olive oil, then with a wire whisk, stir in soy flour, and cook a few minutes until thoroughly blended. Combine half-and-half and water and add slowly to the butter-flour mixture, stirring constantly with the wire whisk. Add salt and pepper to taste. Heat to scalding, then beat in egg yolks, 1 at a time. Do not allow mixture to boil.

17.1 grams of carbohydrate in entire recipe; makes 1 cup of sauce, each tablespoon containing 1.1 grams of carbohydrate.

Spiced Cranberry Sauce

A low-carbohydrate sauce to serve with turkey.

Makes approximately 3 cups

One 1-pound package fresh cranberries
1½ cups water
2 teaspoons freshly grated orange peel
Dash of allspice
Dash of cloves
10 drops orange extract
Artificial sweetener equal to 2 cups sugar

Bring cranberries, water, and orange peel to a boil. Boil until the skin of the berries pops open (about 5 minutes). Remove from heat, add remaining ingredients, and mix till thoroughly combined. Cool in refrigerator before serving.

43.2 grams of carbohydrate in entire recipe; makes approximately 3 cups, each tablespoon containing 0.9 grams of carbohydrate.

Apricot Sauce for Duck or Chicken

Apricot sauce makes a nice change from the usual orange sauce for duck.

Makes approximately 2⅜ cups

2 cups sugar-free, artificially sweetened apricot jam
1 teaspoon minced fresh gingerroot

¼ cup dry sherry
Dash of cardamom
2 dashes cloves
Dash of allspice
2 tablespoons Grand Marnier
⅛ teaspoon minced garlic
Artificial sweetener equal to 1 cup sugar

In a heavy saucepan, combine the jam, gingerroot, sherry, cardamom, cloves, allspice, Grand Marnier, and garlic. Heat over a low flame, stirring frequently until all flavors are thoroughly combined and mixture comes to a boil. Remove from heat and add artificial sweetener. Allow the mixture to stand for 10 to 15 minutes before serving to allow it to thicken again. Spoon the sauce over roasted or barbecued duck or chicken.

177.4 grams of carbohydrate in entire recipe; makes approximately 2⅜ cups of sauce, each tablespoon containing 4.7 grams of carbohydrate.

Blackberry Sauce for Duck or Chicken

A dietetic version of sauce for Duck Montmorency.

Makes approximately 1¼ cups of sauce

1 cup sugar-free, artificially sweetened blackberry jam
1½ teaspoons minced fresh gingerroot
1 tablespoon Cognac or other good brandy
3 tablespoons dry sherry
1 tablespoon fresh lemon juice
Dash of cloves
Dash of cardamom
Dash of coriander
Artificial sweetener equal to 6 tablespoons sugar

In a heavy saucepan, combine the jam, gingerroot, Cognac, sherry, lemon juice, cloves, cardamom, and coriander. Heat over low flame stirring frequently until all flavors are thoroughly combined and mixture comes to a boil. Remove from heat, add artificial sweetener, and wait about 10 minutes before you serve the sauce. This will give the melted liquid a chance to thicken again. Spoon the sauce over roasted or barbecued duck or chicken.

166.2 grams of carbohydrate in entire recipe; makes approximately 1¼ cups of sauce, each tablespoon containing 8.3 grams of carbohydrate.

Mint Jelly

A must for lamb.

Makes approximately 1¾ cups

½ cup fresh mint leaves
1 cup boiling water
1 envelope unflavored gelatin
½ cup cold water
⅓ cup fresh lime juice
Artificial sweetener equal to ¼ cup sugar
4–5 drops green food coloring

Crush mint leaves, then pour boiling water over them. Cover the dish and allow to stand for 5 minutes. Meanwhile, soften the gelatin in cold water for 5 minutes. Strain the mint liquid into the softened gelatin and stir until the gelatin dissolves completely. Add ⅓ cup fresh lime juice, artificial sweetener, and enough green food coloring to make a pretty shade of green. Mix thoroughly, then pour the mixture into a 2-cup mold or pretty serving dish and chill thoroughly.

7.4 grams of carbohydrate in entire recipe; makes approximately 1¾ cups of jelly, each tablespoon containing 0.3 grams of carbohydrate.

Mint Sauce

Try Mint Sauce instead of Mint Jelly with lamb.

Makes approximately 1 cup

1 cup fresh mint leaves
¼ cup boiling water
⅓ cup mild wine vinegar
Artificial sweetener equal to 3 tablespoons sugar

Wash and dry the mint leaves, then chop finely. Place in a bowl and add boiling water. Mix in the vinegar and artificial sweetener. Allow the mixture to stand for at least 2 hours, preferably longer for flavor to develop and blend. Try serving this sauce with lamb chops or leg of lamb, or as a basting sauce when grilling lamb chops or leg of lamb.

4.2 grams of carbohydrate in entire recipe; makes approximately 1 cup of sauce, each tablespoon containing 0.3 grams of carbohydrate.

Curry Sauce for Seafood

This makes a pleasant change from the usual sauces for cold seafood.

Makes 1 cup

¾ cup sugarless mayonnaise
2 tablespoons sour cream, 50 percent reduced fat
2 tablespoons cold water
1 tablespoon Madras curry powder (page 20)
Dash of garlic powder

Combine all ingredients and beat with an electric mixer or a wire whisk until smooth and well blended. Use as a sauce for cold shrimp, lobster, or crabmeat.

9.9 grams of carbohydrate in entire recipe; makes 1 cup of sauce, each tablespoon containing 0.6 grams of carbohydrate.

Dilled Shrimp Sauce

This sauce is the highlight of the meal any time I serve it.

Makes approximately 1 cup

¼ cup sugarless mayonnaise
¼ cup sour cream, 50 percent reduced fat
¼ cup chili sauce
1½ teaspoons freshly grated onion
6 tablespoons chopped fresh dill
Generous dash freshly ground black pepper

Beat the mayonnaise until very smooth and softened. I generally use a glass measuring cup to make this. You measure and make it in the same cup that way. Beat in the sour cream and when thoroughly blended, beat in the chili sauce. Mix in the remaining ingredients in the above order. Allow the sauce to sit for a few hours before serving.

To use as a sauce for shrimp cocktails, arrange fresh, cooked, and cooled shrimp around the dish and place about a tablespoon of the sauce in the center. When used as part of an hors d'oeuvres tray, pour some of the sauce over the shrimp before bringing it to the table. This sauce is also good as a party dip for dipping raw vegetables.

22.2 grams of carbohydrate in entire recipe; makes 1 cup, each tablespoon containing 1.4 grams of carbohydrate.

Garlic and Parsley Sauce for Shrimp

How about cold scampi?

Makes ½ cup

¼ cup olive oil
1½ tablespoons white wine vinegar
1 tablespoon fresh lemon juice
2 tablespoons finely minced parsley, preferably Italian parsley if available
¼ teaspoon salt, or more to taste
⅛ teaspoon dry mustard
1 large clove garlic, minced or put through a press
Generous dash freshly ground black pepper

Combine all ingredients and shake well to blend. Use as a sauce for shrimp cocktails. Arrange the shrimp prettily on a lettuce leaf and spoon some of the sauce over them.

3.2 grams of carbohydrate in entire recipe; makes 8 tablespoons, each tablespoon containing 0.4 grams of carbohydrate.

Mayonnaise Verte

Cold poached salmon without this sauce is nothing.

Makes approximately 2½ cups

2 whole eggs
Juice of 1 lemon
1 large or 2 small cloves of fresh garlic
¾ teaspoon dry mustard
¾ teaspoon salt
2 cups olive oil
¼ cup minced chives, fresh or frozen
20 large spinach leaves, coarsely chopped
¼ cup watercress leaves
½ cup fresh parsley
1 heaping tablespoon fresh tarragon or 2 teaspoons dried tarragon

Place in a blender or food processor the eggs, lemon juice, garlic, dry mustard, and salt. Cover the container and blend at high speed till thoroughly mixed. Remove the feeder cap and slowly add the oil in a steady stream, continuing to run the blender at highest speed. Remove the cover, add the remaining ingredients, re-cover, and continue to blend until all the greens are thoroughly incorporated into the mixture. Remove to a storage container, and chill in refrigerator until serving time.

10 grams of carbohydrate in entire recipe; each tablespoon contains 0.3 grams of carbohydrate.

NOTE: This sauce is marvelous served with cold poached salmon, but can be served deliciously with any cold seafood—

shrimp, lobster, crabmeat, et al. Also, if pasteurized eggs are not available, add garlic, chives, spinach, watercress, and parsley to good store-bought sugar-free mayonnaise.

Creamy Mustard Sauce

A delightful sauce for cold seafood.

Makes 1½ cups

½ cup sugarless mayonnaise
½ cup sour cream, 50 percent reduced fat
¼ cup Dijon-style mustard
¼ cup chopped fresh dill

Beat mayonnaise until very smooth and softened. Beat in the sour cream and when thoroughly blended, beat in the mustard. Fold in the chopped dill. Keep this sauce in the refrigerator for a few hours to blend the flavors and develop them. Use sauce for cold seafood such as shrimp, lobster, scallops, or crabmeat.

18.8 grams of carbohydrate in entire recipe; makes 1½ cups of sauce, each tablespoon containing 0.8 grams of carbohydrate.

Cheese Sauce

Try this cheese sauce over freshly steamed vegetables.

Makes 1 cup

1 recipe White Sauce
¼ cup (1 ounce) grated sharp Cheddar cheese
Dash of cayenne pepper
Dash of nutmeg

Follow ingredients and method for White Sauce (page 251), adding the grated cheese, cayenne pepper, and nutmeg before adding egg yolks. Allow cheese to melt, then beat in the yolks.

17.7 grams of carbohydrate in entire recipe; makes 1 cup of sauce, each tablespoon containing 1.1 grams of carbohydrate.

Vinaigrette Dressing

This is the true French dressing.

Makes 1 cup

¾ cup good-quality olive oil
¼ cup good-quality mild wine vinegar or balsamic vinegar
½ teaspoon salt
Generous sprinkling of freshly ground black pepper
1 clove garlic (optional)

Combine all ingredients in a blender and blend at high speed just until thoroughly combined.

3.0 grams of carbohydrate in entire recipe; makes 1 cup, each tablespoon containing 0.2 grams of carbohydrate.

Beach House Mustard Dressing

This dressing was taught to me by a French girl who visited our beach house in Southampton. It became the favorite of the house.

Makes 1 cup

¼ cup brown mustard
Few dashes of garlic salt
Few dashes of ground celery seed

Few dashes of freshly ground black pepper
¾ cup olive oil
1 tablespoon vinegar

Place the mustard in a medium-size bowl. Add garlic salt, ground celery seed, and pepper. Very slowly with a wire whisk or electric mixer, beat in the oil a little at a time, as if you were making mayonnaise. Do not add more oil until the previous amount is thoroughly blended in or this sauce will curdle. Keep adding oil, mixing it in thoroughly until all oil is used up and the dressing looks like a thick mayonnaise. Beat it in the vinegar to thin it a little. Serve over Salade Niçoise (page 210) or over any tossed green salad.

6.8 grams of carbohydrate in entire recipe; makes 16 tablespoons, each tablespoon containing 0.4 grams of carbohydrate.

Roquefort Dressing

A delight with a green salad.

Makes approximately 1½ cups

¾ cup good-quality olive oil
¼ cup good-quality mild wine vinegar
¼ pound imported French Roquefort cheese, crumbled
Salt and freshly ground pepper to taste

Beat the oil and vinegar until an emulsion is formed. Mash in the Roquefort cheese and mix thoroughly. Add salt and freshly ground black pepper to taste. You can crumble additional Roquefort cheese into the salad if you desire.

5.0 grams of carbohydrate in entire recipe; makes approximately 1½ cups, each tablespoon containing 0.2 grams of carbohydrate.

Cinnamon-Sugar Topping

Use this in place of cinnamon-sugar and you'll barely know the difference.

Makes ½ cup

Granulated sugar substitute, equal to ½ cup sugar
1 teaspoon cinnamon

Mix artificial sweetener and cinnamon until well combined. Store in a glass jar or plastic container to use as desired.

9.1 grams of carbohydrate in entire recipe; makes ½ cup, each teaspoon containing 0.4 grams of carbohydrate.

Pesto Sauce

I like to make my pesto very garlicky. That lets you use less of it with the same results. I love this sauce in everything.

Makes approximately 1 cup of sauce

2 cups torn basil leaves, tightly packed
4 large cloves of fresh garlic, peeled
½ cup extra-virgin olive oil
2 tablespoons pine nuts
½ cup (2 ounces) grated Italian Parmesan cheese
Salt and freshly ground pepper to taste

With the food processor running, drop in the garlic cloves one at a time. Stop the food processor, and add the basil, oil, and the pine nuts. If you are planning to use the sauce immediately, add the cheese, salt, and pepper. If you are not planning on using the sauce immediately, and intend to freeze it for later use, do not add the cheese, salt, and pepper until you are ready to use it. The pesto loses its freshness when you freeze it with the cheese. It will freeze well if you do not add the cheese before freezing.

32.0 grams of carbohydrate in entire recipe; makes 2 cups, each tablespoon containing 1.0 grams of carbohydrate.

Nutted Cheese Spread

Try this with cinnamon bread.

Makes 24 tablespoons

1 8-ounce package whipped cream cheese, light variety
⅓ cup walnuts, coarsely chopped

Allow the cream cheese to stand for about 20 minutes to soften at room temperature. Mix in the walnuts thoroughly. Store in a covered dish in the refrigerator.

18.8 grams of carbohydrate in entire recipe; makes 20 tablespoons, each tablespoon containing 0.9 grams of carbohydrate.

Carbohydrate Gram- and Calorie-Counting Charts

Carbohydrates and Calories
   in Ingredients Used in This Book   268

Carbohydrates and Calories
   in Selected *Low-Carbohydrate* Foods   274

Carbohydrates and Calories
   in Selected *High-Carbohydrate* Foods   280

Carbohydrates and Calories
   in Wines and Other Alcoholic Beverages   288

Carbohydrate Gram- and Calorie-Counting Charts

All foods are not equal in the degree to which they will make you gain weight, even if they have the same carbohydrate and/or calorie values.

A team of doctors, headed by Dr. Walton W. Shreeve at Brookhaven National Laboratory, conducted studies which showed that when patients were fed diets that were alternately high in sugar and starch content, the percentage of sugar converted to blood fat was 2 to 5 percent higher than the percentage of starch converted to blood fat.

This research suggests that any simple carbohydrate food (sugar) is two to five times as fattening as a complex carbohydrate food (starch). Therefore, food containing sugar is two to five times as fattening as food containing starch, even though their carbohydrate gram values may be similar or their calorie amounts equal.

NOTE: Figures in the accompanying charts were compiled from the Department of Agriculture Handbook No. 8, *Composition of Foods* (Washington: United States Department of Agriculture, 1963) and *The Dictionary of Calories & Carbohydrates* by Barbara Kraus (New York: Grosset & Dunlap, 1973). The letters n.d.a. following an entry mean no data available.

Carbohydrates and Calories in Ingredients Used in This Book

**These items are relatively high in carbohydrate value. Use them sparingly.

Food and Quantity	Carbohydrate Grams	Calories
ALMONDS, slivered, 1 tbl.	2.1	63
ANCHOVY PASTE, 1 tbl.	1.0	20
ARTICHOKE HEARTS, frozen, ⅓ pkg.	4.8	22
BACON, cured, broiled or fried crisp, drained		
1 thick slice	0.4	73
1 thin slice	0.2	31
BACON, CANADIAN, unheated, 1 oz.	trace	61
BAKING POWDER, phosphate, 1 teas.	1.4	6
BAMBOO SHOOTS, canned, sliced, ½ cup	1.0	6
BEAN CURD, Chinese, 1 cake (4.2 oz.)	2.9	86
BEAN SPROUTS, canned (La Choy), 1 cup	1.0	15
Fresh, raw, Mung, 4 oz.	7.5	40
Fresh, raw, soy, 4 oz.	6.0	52
BEANS, green or snap, fresh, 4 oz. weighed untrimmed	7.1	32
BEEF		
Flank, raw, 100 percent lean, 4 oz.	0	163
Filet mignon. There are no data available currently, but for the closest possible approximation, use the figures for sirloin steak, lean only.		
Ground, raw, lean, 4 oz.	0	203
Rib steak or roast, roasted or broiled, lean only, boneless, 4 oz.	0	273
Round, raw, lean, 4 oz., boneless	0	249
Steak, sirloin, broiled, lean only, 4 oz.	0	235

Carbohydrate Gram- and Calorie-Counting Charts

Food and Quantity	Carbohydrate Grams	Calories
Steak, T-bone, broiled, lean only, 4 oz.	0	253
**BEETS, canned, solids and liquid, ½ cup	9.7	42
BLUEFISH, raw, meat only, 4 oz.	0	133
BRAZIL NUTS, shelled, ½ cup (2.5 oz.)	7.6	458
BROCCOLI, frozen, spears, ⅓ pkg.	3.6	26
BROTH, beef, canned, 1 cup	2.6	31
BUTTER, 1 tbl.	0.1	100
CABBAGE, white, raw, 4 oz. weighed untrimmed	4.8	22
CABBAGE, Chinese or celery, raw, sliced, ½ cup	1.1	5
CABBAGE, spoon or bok choy, raw, 4 oz. weighed untrimmed	3.2	17
CANTALOUPE, fresh, ¼ of medium-size	7.2	29
**CARAWAY SEEDS, 1 oz.	12.3	72
**CARROT, raw, 5½" × 1"	4.8	21
CAULIFLOWER, fresh, raw, 4 oz. weighed untrimmed	2.3	12
CAULIFLOWER, frozen, ⅓ pkg.	3.2	21
CAVIAR, sturgeon, whole eggs, 1 tbl.	0.5	42
CELERY, raw, diced, ½ cup	2.3	10
CELERY, raw, 1 large outer stalk	1.6	7
CHEESE, 1 oz.		
Blue, natural	0.6	104
Cheddar, natural	0.6	113
Cottage, creamed, unflavored	0.8	30
Cream, plain, unwhipped	0.6	106
Edam, natural	0.3	104
Farmer's	0.6	40
Feta, Greek	trace	100
Mozzarella, made from whole milk	0.8	96
Muenster, natural	0.3	100
Parmesan, natural	0.8	111
Parmesan, natural, grated, 1 tbl.	0.2	31
Pot, uncreamed	0.6	24
Ricotta, Italian style	1.3	50

THE LOW-CARB GOURMET

Food and Quantity	Carbohydrate Grams	Calories
Roquefort, natural	0.6	104
Swiss Emmenthal, natural, imported	0.5	104
Swiss Gruyère, natural, imported	0.5	104
CHICKEN		
Broiler, cooked, meat only, 4 oz.	0	154
Roaster, cooked, dark meat only, 4 oz.	0	209
Roaster, cooked, light meat only, 4 oz.	0	206
CHICKEN BROTH, canned, 1 cup	0.1	30
**CHILI SAUCE, 1 tbl.	3.7	16
CHIVES, raw, 1 oz.	1.6	8
**CHOCOLATE, baking, bitter or unsweetened, 1 oz.	8.2	143
CINNAMON, ground, 1 oz.	25.1	114
CLAM JUICE LIQUOR, bottled or canned, ½ cup	2.5	23
COCOA, dry, unsweetened, Dutch, 1 tbl.	2.9	21
**CORNSTARCH, 1 teas.	2.3	10
**CRANBERRIES fresh, untrimmed, 4 oz.	11.8	50
CREAM, heavy, unwhipped, 1 tbl.	0.5	53
CREAM, sour, 1 tbl.	0.5	25
CUCUMBERS, fresh, eaten without skin, 4 oz. when weighed with skin	2.7	12
CURRY POWDER, 1 teas.	1.3	7
DILL, fresh, probably the same as for PARSLEY	n.d.a.	n.d.a.
DUCK, raw, domesticated, meat and skin, 4 oz.	0	370
DUCK, raw, domesticated, meat only, 4 oz.	0	187
EGGPLANT, whole, 4 oz. weighed untrimmed	5.2	23
EGGS, chicken, raw		
Whole, large	0.4	81
Whole, extra-large	0.5	94
White only, 1, from large egg	0.3	17
Yolk only, 1, from large egg	0.1	59

Carbohydrate Gram- and Calorie-Counting Charts 271

Food and Quantity	Carbohydrate Grams	Calories
ENDIVE, Belgian, raw, 4 oz. weighed untrimmed	3.2	15
ESCAROLE, raw, 4 oz. weighed untrimmed	4.1	20
FLOUR, soybean, full-fat, 1 oz.	4.4	122
**FLOUR, wheat, all-purpose, 1 tbl.	6.8	33
GARLIC, raw, peeled, 1 oz.	8.7	39
GELATIN, unflavored, dry, 1 envelope	0	23
GINGERROOT, fresh, 1 oz. weighed with skin	2.5	13
HAM, boiled, canned, 1 oz.	0.3	55
HAM, Italian prosciutto	n.d.a.	n.d.a.
JAM, artificially sweetened, Louis Sherry, all flavors, 1 jar	3.97	32
JAM, artificially sweetened, all other brands, see label on jar		
LAMB, choice grade, cooked, lean only, leg, 4 oz.	0	211
LEMON JUICE, fresh, 1 tbl.	1.2	4
LEMON PEEL, fresh, raw, 1 oz.	0.4	n.d.a.
LETTUCE, fresh, 4 oz. weighed untrimmed		
Bibb	2.1	12
Boston	2.1	12
Iceberg	3.3	15
Romaine	2.6	13
LIME JUICE, fresh, 1 tbl.	1.3	4
LIVER, calf's, raw, 4 oz.	4.7	159
LIVER, chicken, raw, 4 oz.	3.3	146
LOBSTER, raw, 4 oz. weighed whole	0.6	27
LOBSTER, raw, meat only, 4 oz.	0.6	103
MACKEREL, Spanish, raw, meat only	0	201
MARGARINE, 1 tbl.	0.1	101
MAYONNAISE, Hellmann's or Best Foods, 1 tbl.	0.2	97
MINT, fresh	n.d.a.	n.d.a.
MUSHROOMS, fresh, whole, 4 oz. weighed untrimmed	4.9	31
MUSTARD, prepared, brown, 1 teas.	0.5	8
MUSTARD, prepared, Dijon, 1 teas.	0.4	4

THE LOW-CARB GOURMET

Food and Quantity	Carbohydrate Grams	Calories
OIL, salad or cooking, 1 tbl.		
Olive	0	124
Peanut	0	124
OLIVES,		
Greek style, black, with pits, oil-coated, 1 oz.	2.0	77
Green, pitted and drained, 1 oz.	0.4	33
ONIONS, raw		
Whole, 4 oz. weighed untrimmed	9.0	39
Chopped, 1 tbl.	1.0	4
Grated, 1 tbl.	1.2	5
ORANGE PEEL, raw, 1 oz.	7.1	n.d.a.
PARSLEY, fresh, chopped, 1 tbl.	0.3	2
**PEA PODS, Chinese or edible-podded, snow peas, 4 oz. weighed untrimmed	12.9	57
PECANS, shelled, chopped, 1 tbl.	1.0	48
PEPPER, black, ground, 1 teas.	0.7	4
PEPPERS, sweet, raw		
Green, whole, 4 oz. weighed untrimmed	4.5	21
Green, chopped, 1 tbl.	0.5	2
Red, whole, 4 oz. weighed untrimmed	6.5	28
PORK, fresh, medium fat, 4 oz.		
All lean cuts, boneless, raw	0	210
Ground, lean only, raw	0	210
Spareribs, raw, with bone	0	244
**PUMPKIN, canned, ½ cup	9.6	40
**RASPBERRIES, red, fresh, trimmed, ½ cup	9.8	41
RHUBARB, fresh, 4 oz. weighed untrimmed	1.9	8
ROCK CORNISH HENS	n.d.a.	n.d.a.
	Use figures for CHICKEN	
SALMON, Atlantic, Chinook, or king, fresh, raw meat only, 4 oz.	0	250
SALT, table, 1 teas.	0	0

Carbohydrate Gram- and Calorie-Counting Charts 273

Food and Quantity	Carbohydrate Grams	Calories
SARDINES, skinless and boneless, canned, 1 can weighing 3¾ oz., canned in olive oil	n.d.a.	341
SAUSAGE, pork, Italian style, cooked, 1 oz.	0.3	86
SCALLIONS, green onions, whole, bulb and entire top, 1 oz.	2.3	10
SHAD, raw, meat only, 4 oz.	0	193
SHALLOTS, raw, 1 oz. weighed with skin	4.2	18
SHRIMP, raw, meat only, 4 oz.	1.7	103
SOLE, raw, fillet, meat only, 4 oz.	0	90
SORREL, sour grass, raw, 4 oz. weighed untrimmed	4.5	22
SOYBEAN CURD (see BEAN CURD, Chinese)		
SOY FLOUR, (see FLOUR, soybean, full-fat)		
SOY SAUCE, all-purpose, 1 tbl.	1.4	10
SPINACH, raw, fresh, 4 oz. weighed untrimmed	3.7	21
SQUASH, SUMMER (see ZUCCHINI)		
STRAWBERRIES, fresh, whole, capped, ½ cup	6.1	27
**TOMATO SAUCE, canned, plain, ½ cup	8.4	40
TOMATOES, fresh, ripe, whole with skin, 4 oz.	5.3	25
TOMATOES, canned, regular pack, solids and liquid, ½ cup	5.1	25
TUNA FISH, canned in oil, drained solids, 6½-oz. can	0	309
TURNIPS, fresh, white, without tops, raw, 4 oz. weighed with skins	6.4	29
VANILLA, extract, 1 teas.	n.d.a.	8
VEAL, medium-fat, raw, boneless, leg, lean meat only, 4 oz.	0	205
VINEGAR, distilled, 1 tbl.	0.8	2
WALNUTS, English or Persian, shelled, chopped, 1 tbl.	1.2	49

Food and Quantity	Carbohydrate Grams	Calories
**WATER CHESTNUTS, fresh, raw, whole, 4 oz. weighed unpeeled	16.6	68
WATERCRESS raw, 4 oz. weighed untrimmed	3.1	20
WATERCRESS raw, trimmed, ½ cup	0.5	3
**WORCESTERSHIRE SAUCE, 1 tbl.		
Lea & Perrins	3.0	12
French's	1.4	6
ZUCCHINI, green, fresh, raw, 4 oz. weighed untrimmed	3.9	18

Carbohydrates and Calories in Selected *Low-Carbohydrate* Foods

This is a list of foods that low-carbohydrate dieters should concentrate on. The starred (**) items are slightly higher in carbohydrates, but are nevertheless good for dieters if used in moderation.

Food and Quantity	Carbohydrate Grams	Calories
ABALONE, canned, 4 oz.	2.6	91
ALBACORE, raw, meat only, 4 oz.	0	201
ANCHOVY PASTE, 1 tbl.	1.0	20
APRICOT, fresh, whole, 1 if 12 per pound	4.6	18
ASPARAGUS, fresh, 4 oz. weighed untrimmed	3.2	17
AVOCADO, peeled, pitted		
California variety, ½ cup cubes	4.6	130
Florida variety, ½ cup cubes	6.7	97
BASS, black sea, raw, weighed whole, 1 lb.	0	119
BASS, striped, raw, meat only, 4 oz.	0	165
BEANS, yellow or wax, cooked and drained, 4 oz.	5.2	25

Carbohydrate Gram- and Calorie-Counting Charts

Food and Quantity	Carbohydrate Grams	Calories
BEEF, chipped, uncooked, ½ cup	0	166
BEET GREENS, fresh, raw whole, 4 oz. weighed untrimmed	2.9	15
**BLACKBERRIES (including boysenberries, dewberries, and youngberries), fresh, hulled, ½ cup	9.4	42
BLOOD PUDDING or sausage, 1 oz.	0.1	112
**BLUEBERRIES, fresh, trimmed, ½ cup	11.2	45
BOLOGNA, all-meat, 1 oz.	1.0	79
BONITO, raw, meat only, 4 oz.	0	191
BROAD BEANS, Italian, frozen, ⅓ pkg.	4.1	23
BROCCOLI, fresh, raw, whole, 4 oz. weighed untrimmed	4.1	22
**BRUSSELS SPROUTS, fresh, raw, 4 oz. weighed untrimmed	8.7	47
CABBAGE, spoon, white mustard, or bok choy, fresh, raw, 4 oz. weighed untrimmed	3.2	17
CAPERS, 1 tbl.	1.0	6
CARP, raw, meat only, 4 oz.	0	130
CASABA MELON, fresh, flesh only, 4 oz.	7.4	31
CERVELAT, 1 oz.		
Dry	0.5	128
Soft	0.5	87
CHARD, Swiss, fresh, raw, whole, 4 oz. weighed untrimmed	4.8	26
CHEWING GUM, Bazooka, bubble, sugarless, 1 piece	trace	16
Care Free (Beech Nut), sugarless, 1 stick	trace	6
CHICORY GREENS, fresh, raw, 4 oz. weighed untrimmed	3.5	19
CLAMS, all kinds, raw, meat only, 3 oz.	1.7	65
Canned, meat only, ½ cup	1.5	78
**COCONUT, fresh, meat only, 4 oz.	10.7	392
**COCONUT CREAM, liquid expressed from grated coconut, 4 oz.	9.4	379

THE LOW-CARB GOURMET

Food and Quantity	Carbohydrate Grams	Calories
COCONUT MILK, liquid expressed from a mixture of grated coconut and water, 4 oz.	5.9	286
COD, raw, meat only, 4 oz.	0	88
COLLARD GREENS, fresh, raw, leaves only, 4 oz.	5.8	35
CONSOMMÉ MADRILÈNE, canned, Crosse & Blackwell, ½ can	2.4	33
CORNED BEEF, cooked, boneless, medium-fat, 4 oz.	0	422
CRAB, all species, steamed		
Whole, 4 oz. weighed in shell	0.3	51
Meat only, 1 cup (4.4 oz.)	0.6	116
EGG BEATERS, Fleischmann's, ¼ cup	0.5	100
FENNEL, raw, 4 oz. weighed untrimmed	5.4	30
FILBERTS, shelled, 1 oz.	4.7	180
FLOUNDER, raw, meat only, 4 oz.	0	90
FRANKFURTER, all-beef, 6 oz.	1.1	134
GELATIN DESSERT, dietetic, D-Zerta, all flavors, ½ cup	trace	8
GOOSE, domesticated, roasted, meat and skin, 4 oz.	0	500
**GRAPEFRUIT, fresh, seedless, pulp only		
White, ½ medium-size (8.5 oz.)	11.9	44
Pink and red, ½ medium-size, (8.5 oz.)	12.8	49
**GRAPES, Fresh, American type, Concord, Delaware, Niagara, Catawba, and scuppernong, 4 oz. weighed untrimmed	11.2	49
GROUPER, raw, meat only, 4 oz.	0	99
HADDOCK, raw, meat only, 4 oz.	0	90
HAKE, raw, meat only, 4 oz.	0	84
HALIBUT, all varieties, raw, meat only, 4 oz.	0	113
HEADCHEESE, 1 oz.	0.3	76
HERRING, kippered, smoked, 4 oz.	0	239
HICKORY NUTS, shelled, 1 oz.	3.6	191

Carbohydrate Gram- and Calorie-Counting Charts 277

Food and Quantity	Carbohydrate Grams	Calories
HONEYDEW MELON, fresh, flesh only, 4 oz.	8.7	37
HORSERADISH, raw, pared, 1 oz.	5.6	25
HORSERADISH, prepared, 1 oz.	2.7	11
KALE, raw, leaves only, 4 oz. weighed untrimmed	6.5	39
KIDNEY, beef, raw, 4 oz.	1.0	147
KIDNEY, lamb, raw, 4 oz.	1.0	119
KINGFISH, raw, meat only, 4 oz.	0	119
KNOCKWURST, all-beef, 1 oz.	0.6	79
KOHLRABI, raw, whole, weighed with skin, without leaves, 4 oz.	5.5	24
LAKE TROUT, raw, meat only, 4 oz.	0	191
**LITCHI NUTS, fresh, whole, 4 oz. weighed in shell with seeds	11.2	44
LIVER SAUSAGE or LIVERWURST, 1 oz.	0.5	87
MANDARIN ORANGES, canned, unsweetened, solids and liquids, 4 oz.	7.1	31
**MANGO, fresh, whole, 4 oz. weighed with seeds and skin	12.8	50
MAPLE SYRUP, dietetic (Tillie Lewis), 1 tbl.	0.9	3
**MILK, dry, nonfat, instant (Carnation), ¼ cup powder	9.4	61
**MILK, fresh, 1 cup		
Whole, 3.5 percent fat	12.0	159
Skimmed	12.5	88
Buttermilk, cultured	12.5	88
MORTADELLA, sausage, 1 oz.	0.2	89
MULLET, raw, meat only, 4 oz.	0	166
MUSSELS, Atlantic and Pacific, meat only, 4 oz.	3.7	108
MUSTARD GREENS, raw, whole, 4 oz. weighed untrimmed	4.5	25
OCEAN PERCH, raw, meat only, 4 oz.	0	108
OCTOPUS, raw, meat only, 4 oz.	0	83

278 THE LOW-CARB GOURMET

Food and Quantity	Carbohydrate Grams	Calories
OKRA, raw, whole, 4 oz. weighed untrimmed	7.7	35
OYSTERS, Eastern, meat only, 4 oz.	3.9	75
OYSTERS, Pacific and Western, meat only, 4 oz.	7.3	103
**PAPAYA, fresh, flesh only, 4 oz.	11.3	44
PÂTÉ DE FOIE GRAS, canned, 1 oz.	1.4	131
**PEACHES, fresh, whole, 4 oz. weighed unpeeled	9.6	38
PEANUT BUTTER, 1 tbl.		
Skippy, chunk or creamy	2.3	102
Smucker's, creamy or crunchy	2.4	85
Smucker's, old-fashioned	1.6	85
PHEASANT, raw, meat and skin, 4 oz.	0	172
PICKLES, dill, 4" × 1¾"	3.0	15
PICKLES, cucumber, 4" × 1¾"	2.7	14
PIKE, raw, meat only, 4 oz.	0	102
PIMENTO, canned, solids and liquids, 1 med.	2.2	10
**PINEAPPLE, fresh, raw, whole, 4 oz. weighed untrimmed	8.1	31
POLLACK, raw, meat only, 4 oz.	0	108
POMPANO, raw, meat only, 4 oz.	0	188
PORGY, raw, meat only, 4 oz.	0	127
PORK SAUSAGE, all-meat (Jones), 1 oz.	0	n.d.a.
RADISHES, common or Oriental, raw, untrimmed without tops, 4 oz.	3.7	17
RED or GRAY SNAPPER, raw, meat only, 4 oz.	0	105
ROCKFISH, raw, meat only, 4 oz.	0	110
ROE, SHAD, raw, 4 oz.	1.7	147
**RUTABAGA, raw, diced, ½ cup	7.7	32
SABLEFISH, raw, meat only, 4 oz.	0	215
SALAMI, all-meat, cooked, 1 oz.	0.4	88
SALAMI, all-meat, dry, 1 oz.	0.3	128
SAND DABS, raw, meat only, 4 oz.	0	90
SALT PORK, without skin, 1 oz.	0	222

Carbohydrate Gram- and Calorie-Counting Charts 279

Food and Quantity	Carbohydrate Grams	Calories
TARTAR SAUCE, Hellmann's or Best Foods, 1 tbl.	0.3	73
SAUERKRAUT, canned, drained solids, ½ cup	3.1	16
SCALLOPS, raw, muscle only, 4 oz.	3.7	92
SESAME SEEDS, dry		
Hulled, 1 oz.	5.0	165
Whole, 1 oz.	6.1	160
SESAME SEEDS, liquid, tahini (A. Sahadi), 1 tbl.	0.8	57
SKATE, raw, meat only, 4 oz.	0	111
SMELTS, all kinds, raw, meat only, 4 oz.	0	111
SNAILS, giant African, 4 oz.	5.0	83
SNAILS, raw, 4 oz.	2.3	102
SOYBEAN MILK, fluid, 4 oz.	2.5	37
SQUAB, pigeon, raw, meat and skin, 4 oz.	0	333
SQUASH, summer, crookneck and straight neck, yellow, fresh, raw, 4 oz. weighed untrimmed	4.8	22
STURGEON, smoked, meat only, 4 oz.	0	169
SWEETBREADS, calf, raw, 4 oz.	0	102
SWORDFISH, raw, meat only, 4 oz.	0	134
**TANGERINES, whole, 4 oz. weighed untrimmed	9.7	39
TOMATO JUICE, canned, reg. pack, ½ cup	5.2	23
**TOMATO PASTE, 1 tbl.	3.0	13
TONGUE, beef, med. fat, braised, 4 oz.	0.5	277
TROUT, brook, fresh, raw, meat only, 4 oz.	0	115
TURBOT, Greenland, raw, meat only, 4 oz.	0	166
TURNIP GREENS, fresh, raw, 4 oz. weighed untrimmed	4.8	27
VEGETABLE JUICE COCKTAIL, canned, 4 oz.	4.1	19
WHITEFISH, lake, raw, meat only, 4 oz.	0	176
YEAST, baker's		
Compressed, 1 oz.	3.1	24
Dry, 1 pkg.	2.7	20

Food and Quantity	Carbohydrate Grams	Calories
**YOGURT, unflavored		
Made from whole milk, 1 cup	12.6	122
Made from partially skimmed milk, 8 oz.	11.8	113

Carbohydrates and Calories in Selected *High-Carbohydrate* Foods

These are foods low-carbohydrate dieters should avoid.

Food and Quantity	Carbohydrate Grams	Calories
ANGEL FOOD CAKE, home recipe, 1/12 of 8" cake	24.1	108
ANGEL FOOD CAKE MIX, prepared as directed, 1/12 of 10" cake	31.5	137
APPLE, dried, uncooked, ½ cup (1½ oz.)	27.3	106
APPLE, fresh, eaten with skin, 4 oz. weighed untrimmed	15.1	61
APPLE BUTTER, 1 tbl.	8.4	33
APPLE CIDER, ½ cup	14.8	58
APPLE JUICE, canned, ½ cup	14.8	58
APPLE PIE, 2-crust, home recipe, 1/6 of 9" pie	60.2	404
APPLESAUCE, canned, sweetened with sugar, ½ cup	30.5	116
APPLE TURNOVER, frozen	30.2	315
APRICOTS, canned, sweetened with sugar, heavy syrup, halves and syrup, ½ cup	27.7	108
BAGEL, egg, 3" dia.	28.0	165
BAGEL, water, 3" dia.	30.0	165
BANANA PIE, cream or custard, home recipe, 1/6 of 9" pie	46.7	336
BANANAS common, fresh, medium-size, 6.2 oz.	26.4	101

Carbohydrate Gram- and Calorie-Counting Charts

Food and Quantity	Carbohydrate Grams	Calories
BARLEY, pearlized, dry, ½ cup	78.8	348
BEANS, baked, 1 cup		
Canned in pork and molasses sauce	53.8	382
Canned with tomato sauce	58.6	306
Canned with pork and tomato sauce	48.4	311
BEANS, kidney or red, dry, 4 oz.	70.2	389
BEANS, lima		
Young, raw, without shell, 4 oz.	25.1	140
Young, cooked, ½ cup	16.8	94
Mature, dry, baby, ½ cup	61.4	331
BEANS, pinto, dry, ½ cup	61.2	335
BEANS, red, Mexican, 4 oz.	72.2	396
BEANS, white, dry, raw, navy or pea, ½ cup	63.8	354
BEEF PIE, home recipe, 4¼" dia., 8 oz. before baking	42.7	558
BISCUIT, baking powder, home recipe, 2" dia., 1 oz. biscuit	12.8	103
BLUEBERRY PIE, home recipe, 2-crust, ⅙ of 9" pie	55.1	382
BOSTON CREAM PIE, home recipe, 1/12 of 8" pie	34.4	208
BRAN FLAKES, raisin, ½ cup	19.8	72
BREAD		
Boston brown, 1.7 oz. slice, 3" × ¾"	21.9	101
Pumpernickel, 0.8 oz. slice, 20 slices per lb.	12.2	57
Raisin, 0.9 oz. slice, 18 slices per lb.	13.4	66
Rye, light, 0.9 oz. slice, 18 slices per lb.	13.0	61
White, enriched or unenriched, 0.8 oz. slice	11.6	62
Whole wheat, prepared with water, 0.9 oz. slice	12.3	60
BREAD CRUMBS, dry, grated, ½ cup	36.7	196
BREADFRUIT, fresh, peeled and trimmed, 4 oz.	29.7	117

282   THE LOW-CARB GOURMET

Food and Quantity	Carbohydrate Grams	Calories
BUCKWHEAT, groats, kasha, 1 oz.	23.3	108
BULGUR, dry, from hard, red, winter wheat, 4 oz.	85.9	401
CANDY[1]		
CASHEW NUTS, ½ cup	20.5	393
CHERRIES		
Sour, canned, pitted, in heavy syrup, ½ cup	29.5	116
Sweet, fresh, whole, 4 oz. weighed with stems	17.8	72
Sweet, canned, pitted, in heavy syrup, 4 oz.	23.2	92
CHERRY PIE, home recipe, 2-crust, ⅙ of 9" pie	60.7	412
CHESTNUTS, fresh, 4 oz. weighed in shell	38.7	178
CHEWING GUM, sweetened with sugar, 1 stick	2.9	10
CHICKPEAS or GARBANZOS, dry, ½ cup	61.0	360
CHILI CON CARNE, canned, with beans, 1 cup	30.5	332
CHOCOLATE CAKE, without icing, 3 oz.	44.2	311
CHOCOLATE CAKE, 2-layer, with icing, 1/16 of 10" cake	67.0	443
CHOCOLATE CHIFFON PIE, home recipe, ⅙ of 9" pie	61.2	459
CHOCOLATE MERINGUE PIE, home recipe, ⅙ of 9" pie	46.9	353
CHOCOLATE PUDDING, sweetened with sugar, prepared with milk, ½ cup	29.6	161

[1] Under no circumstances can I advocate eating either candy or cookies when one is dieting. Neither has any nutritional value. However, if you are determined, check Barbara Kraus's *A Dictionary of Calories and Carbohydrates* for a complete listing of brand-name candy and cookies and choose ones with the least carbohydrates. Also, see my sweets recipes in Chapter II of this book.

Carbohydrate Gram- and Calorie-Counting Charts

Food and Quantity	Carbohydrate Grams	Calories
CHOCOLATE SYRUP, sweetened with sugar, fudge type, 1 tbl.	10.3	63
CHOCOLATE SYRUP, Hershey's, 1 tbl.	16.7	69
CHUTNEY, 1 tbl.	13.1	53
CITRON, candied, 1 oz.	22.7	89
COCOA MIX, with nonfat dry milk, 1 oz.	20.1	102
COCOA MIX, without nonfat dry milk, 1 oz.	25.3	98
COCONUT, dried, canned or pkg., sweetened, shredded, ½ cup lightly packed	24.5	252
COCONUT CUSTARD PIE, home recipe, ⅙ of 9" pie	37.8	357
CORN, fresh, white or yellow, raw, on cob, husk removed, 8 oz.	27.6	120
CORN, fresh, white or yellow, raw, kernels, 4 oz.	25.1	109
CORN, canned, cream style, white or yellow, reg. pkg., ½ cup	25.0	102
CORN FLAKES, cereal, whole, 1 cup (1 oz.)	24.7	112
CORN SYRUP, light or dark blend, 1 tbl.	15.8	61
CORNBREAD, Southern style, home recipe, prepared with whole ground corn meal, 4 oz.	33.0	235
CORNMEAL, white or yellow, dry, degermed, ½ cup	54.1	251
CRACKER MEAL, ½ cup	56.8	352
CRANBERRY SAUCE, canned, sweetened with sugar, strained, ½ cup	51.0	199
CUPCAKE, home recipe, 2¾" dia., with chocolate icing	29.7	184
CUSTARD APPLE, fresh, flesh only, 4 oz.	28.6	115
DATES, dry, 4 oz. weighed with pits	71.9	270
DOUGHNUT, cake type, 1 piece (1.1 oz.)	16.4	125
ÉCLAIR, home recipe, custard filling and chocolate icing, 4 oz.	26.3	271
FARINA, regular, dry, ½ cup	65.1	314

THE LOW-CARB GOURMET

Food and Quantity	Carbohydrate Grams	Calories
FIGS, fresh, 4 oz.	23	91
FLOUR		
Carob or St. John's bread, 1 oz.	22.9	51
Chestnut, 1 oz.	21.6	103
Rye, med., 1 oz.	21.2	99
Wheat, all-purpose, 1 oz.	21.6	103
Whole wheat, 1 oz.	20.1	94
FRUIT COCKTAIL, canned, packed in heavy syrup, solids and liquid, ½ cup	25.2	97
GELATIN DESSERT, powder, regular, dry, all flavors, 3 oz. pkg.	74.8	315
GINGER, candied, 1 oz.	24.7	96
GINGERBREAD, home recipe, 2" × 2" × 2"	28.6	174
GRAPE JUICE, canned, ½ cup	20.9	83
HONEY, strained, 1 tbl.	16.5	61
ICE CREAM, sweetened with sugar		
10 percent fat, reg. or French, 1 cup	27.7	257
12 percent fat, 1 cup	29.3	294
16 percent fat, rich, 1 cup	26.6	329
Chocolate, Sealtest, ¼ pt.	17.3	136
Vanilla, Lady Borden, 14 percent fat, ¼ pt.	17.0	162
Fudge Royale, Sealtest, ¼ pt.	18.2	132
Strawberry, Sealtest, ¼ pt.	19.5	133
ICE MILK, soft-serve, ½ cup	19.6	133
JAM, sweetened with sugar, 1 tbl.	14.0	54
JELLY, sweetened with sugar, 1 tbl.	12.7	49
JERUSALEM ARTICHOKES, 4 oz. weighed untrimmed	13.1	52
JUJUBE or Chinese dates, fresh, whole, 4 oz. weighed with seeds	29.1	111
KUMQUATS, fresh, 4 oz. weighed with seeds	18.0	69
LEMONADE, frozen concentrate, sweetened with sugar, 6 fl. oz. can	112.0	427

Carbohydrate Gram- and Calorie-Counting Charts 285

Food and Quantity	Carbohydrate Grams	Calories
LEMON MERINGUE PIE, home recipe, 1-crust, ⅙ of 9" pie	52.8	357
LENTILS, whole, dry, 4 oz.	68.2	386
LOGANBERRIES, fresh, 4 oz. weighed with caps	16.1	67
MACARONI, dry, 1 oz.	21.3	105
MALTED MILK MIX, dry, powder, unfortified, 1 oz.	20.1	116
MAPLE SYRUP, 1 tbl.	13.0	50
MARMALADE, sweetened with sugar, 1 tbl.	14.0	51
MATZO MEAL (Manischewitz), ½ cup	48.1	219
MATZOS, regular (Manischewitz), 1 matzo	28.1	114
MILK, CONDENSED, sweetened, canned, 1 cup	166.2	982
MINCE PIE, home recipe, 2-crust, ⅙ of 9" pie	65.1	428
MOLASSES, Barbados, 1 tbl.	13.3	51
MOLASSES, blackstrap, 1 tbl.	10.4	40
MUFFINS		
Blueberry, home recipe, 3" muffin (1.4 oz.)	16.8	112
Bran, home recipe, 3" muffin, (1.4 oz.)	17.2	104
Corn, home recipe, 3" muffin (1.4 oz.)	19.2	126
English, Thomas's, 1 muffin	28.4	140
NECTARINES, fresh, flesh only, 4 oz.	19.4	73
NOODLES, dry, 1½" strips, 1 cup	52.6	283
NOODLES, chow mein, canned, 1 cup	26.1	220
OATMEAL, regular, dry, ½ cup	24.6	141
ORANGES, fresh, whole, medium-size, 3" dia. (5.5 oz.)	19.0	77
ORANGE PEEL, candied, 1 oz.	22.9	90
PANCAKES, home recipe, wheat, 1 4" pancake	9.2	62
PASTINAS, dry, egg, 1 oz.	20.4	109

THE LOW-CARB GOURMET

Food and Quantity	Carbohydrate Grams	Calories
PEAS, mature seeds, dry, split, without seed coat, ½ cup	63.7	353
PEA SOUP, canned, green, prepared with equal volume of water, 1 cup	22.5	130
PEARS, fresh, whole, 4 oz. weighed untrimmed	15.8	63
PICKLES, cucumber, bread and butter, ½ cup	15.2	62
PICKLES, cucumber, sweet, whole, 1 oz.	10.3	41
PIE CRUST, home recipe, baked for 9" pie, 1-crust	78.8	900
PINEAPPLE JUICE, canned, unsweetened, ½ cup	16.7	68
PIZZA, frozen, baked, ⅛ of 14" pie	26.6	184
PLANTAINS, raw, flesh only, 4 oz.	35.4	135
PLUMS, Damson, fresh, whole, 4 oz. weighed with pits	18.4	68
POTATO CHIPS, 1 oz.	21.5	111
POTATO SALAD, home recipe, made with mayonnaise, hard-cooked egg, and seasonings, ½ cup	16.8	181
POTATOES, raw, whole, 4 oz. weighed unpared	15.7	70
POTATOES, french-fried in deep fat, 10 pieces, each 2" × ½" × ½"	20.5	156
PRETZELS, 1 oz.	21.5	111
PRUNES, dried, "softenized," uncooked, medium-size, whole, with pits, ½ cup	53.6	203
PRUNES, canned, stewed, pitted (Del Monte), ½ cup	37.5	144
PRUNE JUICE, ½ cup	24.3	99
PUMPKIN PIE, home recipe, 1-crust, ⅙ of 9" pie	37.2	321
RAISINS, dried, whole, 4 oz.	87.8	328
RICE		
Brown, cooked, 4 oz.	28.9	135
White, regular, raw, ½ cup.	79.6	359

Carbohydrate Gram- and Calorie-Counting Charts

Food and Quantity	Carbohydrate Grams	Calories
White, regular, cooked, ½ cup	24.7	111
SHERBET, orange, ½ cup	29.7	130
SODA, sweetened with sugar, all flavors[2]		
SPAGHETTI, dry, 1 oz.	21.3	105
SPONGE CAKE, home recipe, 1/12 of 10" cake	35.7	196
SQUASH, butternut, baked, flesh only, 4 oz.	19.8	77
SUCCOTASH, frozen, cooked, drained, ½ cup	19.7	89
SUGAR		
Brown, 1 tbl.	12.5	48
Confectioner's, 1 tbl. unsifted	7.7	30
Granulated, 1 tbl.	11.9	46
SWEET POTATOES, raw, all kinds, 4 oz. weighed with skin	24.2	105
TAPIOCA, dry, quick-cooking granulated, ¼ cup	32.8	134
WAFFLES, home recipe, 7" dia. (2.6 oz.)	28.1	209
WATERMELON, fresh, wedge, 2 lbs., 4" × 8" with rind	27.3	111
YAMS, raw, 4 oz. weighed with skin	22.6	99
YOGURT[3]		

---

[2] All soda sweetened with sugar is much too high in carbohydrates for any dieter to use. Six ounces of the average sugar-sweetened soda contain approximately 20 grams of carbohydrates and approximately 80 calories—neither of which have any nutritional value.

[3] All flavored yogurt, no matter which brand or flavor, is high in carbohydrates and should be avoided.

Carbohydrates and Calories in Wines and Other Alcoholic Beverages

Even though these charts are accurate as far as exact carbohydrate and calorie values are concerned, they do not and cannot take into account the effect of alcohol on the body.

Alcohol makes the body produce insulin. Since one of the normal functions of insulin is to convert carbohydrates into fat, anything that increases the insulin level will fatten you faster. At the same time, the effect of alcohol varies from one individual to another. So, despite the fact that exact carbohydrate values are shown here, a dieter should experiment and adjust his alcoholic intake according to what it does to him in particular. No hard and fast rules can be drawn.

Assorted Alcoholic Beverages

Food and Quantity	Carbohydrate Grams	Calories
ANISETTE		
Garnier, 54 proof, 1 oz.	9.3	82
Old Mr. Boston, 60 proof, 1 oz.	7.5	90
B & B LIQUEUR, 86 proof, 1 fl. oz.	5.7	94
BEER		
Regular, 4.5% alcohol, 12 fl. oz.	13.7	151
Lo Carbo Dia Beer, 12 fl. oz.	4.2	145
BITTER LEMON, 6 fl. oz.	23.6	96
BITTER ORANGE, 6 fl. oz.	22.6	92
BITTERS, Angostura, 1 fl. oz.	12.5	86
CHERRY HEERING, liqueur (Hiram Walker), 49 proof, 1 fl. oz.	10.0	80
CHERRIES, MARASCHINO, 1 average cherry	1.9	8
CRÈME DE CASSIS LIQUEUR, Garnier, 60 proof, 1 fl. oz.	13.5	83
CURAÇAO LIQUEUR, Garnier, 60 proof, 1 fl. oz.	12.7	100

Carbohydrate Gram- and Calorie-Counting Charts 289

Food and Quantity	Carbohydrate Grams	Calories
DAIQUIRI COCKTAIL		
Liquid mix, Party Tyme, 2 fl. oz.	19.4	81
Liquid mix, Party Tyme, banana, 2 fl. oz.	14.6	59
DISTILLED LIQUOR, unflavored bourbon whiskey, brandy, Canadian whiskey, gin, Irish whiskey, rum, rye whiskey, Scotch whiskey, tequila, and vodka		
80 proof, 1 fl. oz.	trace	65
86 proof, 1 fl. oz.	trace	70
90 proof, 1 fl. oz.	trace	74
94 proof, 1 fl. oz.	trace	77
100 proof, 1 fl. oz.	trace	83
DRAMBUIE LIQUEUR, 80 proof, Hiram Walker, 1 fl.oz.	11.0	110
GIN, sloe, Garnier, 60 proof, 1 fl. oz.	8.5	83
KIRSCHWASSER, Leroux, 96 proof, 1 fl. oz.	0	80
MANHATTAN COCKTAIL, Hiram Walker, 55 proof, 3 fl. oz.	3.0	147
MARTINI COCKTAIL		
Gin, Hiram Walker, 67.5 proof, 3 fl. oz.	0.6	168
Vodka, Hiram Walker, 60 proof, 3 fl. oz.	0	147
OLD-FASHIONED, Hiram Walker, 62 proof, 3 fl.oz.	3.0	165
PIÑA COLADA, Party Tyme, canned, 12.5% alcohol, 2 fl. oz.	5.1	63
QUININE TONIC WATER, sweetened with sugar		
Canada Dry, 6 fl. oz.	17.6	68
Schweppes, 6 fl. oz.	16.5	66
QUININE TONIC WATER, artificially sweetened, dietetic No-Cal, 6 fl. oz.	0	2
TIA MARIA, liqueur, Hiram Walker, 63 proof, 1 fl. oz.	10.0	92
TOM COLLINS, canned, Party Tyme, 10% alcohol, 2 fl. oz.	5.9	58
TOM COLLINS MIXER SOFT DRINK		
Canada Dry, 6 fl.oz.	15.0	61
Hoffman, 6 fl. oz.	16.1	64

290 THE LOW-CARB GOURMET

Food and Quantity	Carbohydrate Grams	Calories
TRIPLE SEC LIQUEUR, Garnier, 60 proof, 1 fl. oz.	8.5	83
VERMOUTH, dry and extra dry, Noilly Prat, 16% alcohol 3 fl. oz.	1.6	101
VERMOUTH, sweet, Noilly Prat, 16% alcohol, 3 fl. oz.	12.1	128
VODKA SCREWDRIVER, Old Mr. Boston, 25 proof, 3 fl. oz.	10.5	117
WHISKEY SOUR, canned, Hiram Walker, 3 fl. oz.	12.0	177

Wines

BEAUJOLAIS, French, Burgundy		
Barton & Guestier, St. Louis, 12% alcohol, 3 fl. oz.	0.1	60
Chanson, St. Vincent, 11% alcohol, 3 fl. oz.	6.3	84
BURGUNDY		
Gallo, 13% alcohol, 3 fl. oz.	0.9	52
Louis M. Martini, 12.5% alcohol, 3 fl. oz.	0.2	90
BURGUNDY, SPARKLING		
Barton & Guestier, French red, 12% alcohol, 3 fl. oz.	2.2	69
Chanson, French red, 3 fl. oz.	3.6	72
Taylor, 12.5% alcohol, 3 fl. oz.	1.8	78
CHABLIS		
Barton & Guestier, 12% alcohol, 3 fl. oz.	0.1	60
Chanson, St. Vincent, 11.5% alcohol, 3 fl. oz.	6.3	81
Gallo, 12% alcohol, 3 fl. oz.	0.9	50
Louis M. Martini, 12.5% alcohol, 3 fl. oz.	0.2	90
CHAMPAGNE		
Bollinger, 3 fl. oz.	3.6	72
Mumm's Cordon Rouge, brut, 12%, 3 fl. oz.	1.4	65

Carbohydrate Gram- and Calorie-Counting Charts 291

Food and Quantity	Carbohydrate Grams	Calories
Veuve Clicquot, 12.5% alcohol, 3 fl. oz.	0.6	78
CHÂTEAUNEUF-DU-PAPE		
Barton & Guestier, 13.5% alcohol, 3 fl. oz.	0.5	70
Chanson, 13% alcohol, 3 fl. oz.	6.3	90
CHIANTI		
Antinori, Classico, 12.5% alcohol, 3 fl. oz.	6.3	87
Brolio Classico, 13% alcohol, 3 fl. oz.	0.3	66
CLARET		
Gold Seal, 12% alcohol, 3 fl. oz.	0.4	82
COLD DUCK		
Italian Swiss Colony—Private Stock, 12.5% alcohol, 3 fl. oz.	4.3	75
CONCORD WINE		
Mogen David, 12% alcohol, 3 fl. oz.	16.0	120
GEWÜRZTRAMINER		
Willm Alsatian, 11–14% alcohol, 3 fl. oz.	3.6	66
MADEIRA		
Leacock, 19% alcohol, 3 fl. oz.	6.3	120
MARGAUX, French red Bordeaux		
Barton & Guestier, 12% alcohol, 3 fl. oz.	0.4	62
MARSALA		
Italian Swiss Colony—Private Stock, 19.7% alcohol, 3 fl. oz.	7.1	124
PINOT CHARDONNAY		
Louis M. Martini, 12.5% alcohol, 3 fl. oz.	0.2	90
PORT		
Gallo, ruby, 20% alcohol, 3 fl. oz.	8.8	112
Robertson, ruby, 20% alcohol, 3 fl. oz.	9.9	138
Robertson, tawny, 21% alcohol, 3 fl. oz.	9.9	145
POUILLY-FUISSÉ, French white Burgundy		
Barton & Guestier, 12.5% alcohol, 3 fl. oz.	0.3	64
Chanson, St. Vincent, 12% alcohol, 3 fl. oz.	6.3	84

THE LOW-CARB GOURMET

Food and Quantity	Carbohydrate Grams	Calories
POUILLY-FUMÉ, French white, Loire Valley		
Barton & Guestier, 12% alcohol, 3 fl. oz.	0.1	60
RIESLING, Alsatian		
Willm, 11–14% alcohol, 3 fl. oz.	3.6	66
ROSÉ		
Chanson Rosé des Anges, 12% alcohol, 3 fl. oz.	6.3	84
Nectarose, Vin Rosé d'Anjou, 12% alcohol, 3 fl. oz.	2.6	70
ROSÉ, SPARKLING		
Chanson, 3 fl. oz.	3.6	72
SAINT-ÉMILION, French Bordeaux		
Barton & Guestier, 12% alcohol, 3 fl. oz.	0.7	63
SAUTERNES, French white Bordeaux		
Barton & Guestier, 13% alcohol, 3 fl. oz.	7.6	95
SHERRY, CREAM		
Gallo, 20% alcohol, 3 fl. oz.	8.3	111
Williams & Humbert, Canasta, 20.5% alcohol, 3 fl. oz.	5.4	150
SHERRY, DRY		
Dry Sack, Williams & Humbert, 20.5% alcohol, 3 fl. oz.	4.5	120
Gallo, 20% alcohol, 3 fl. oz.	1.7	84
SHERRY, MEDIUM		
Italian Swiss Colony—Private Label, 19.8% alcohol, 3 fl.oz.	2.8	108
Taylor, 19.5% alcohol, 3 fl. oz.	7.1	132
SOAVE, Italian white		
Antinori, 12% alcohol, 3 fl. oz.	6.3	84
SYLVANER		
Louis M. Martini, 12.5% alcohol, 3 fl. oz.	0.2	90
VALPOLICELLA, Italian red		
Antinori, 3 fl. oz.	6.3	84

Index

Agatston, Dr. Arthur, *South Beach Diet Good Fats, Good Carbs Guide,* 9
Air Force Diet, The (Drinking Man's Diet), 6
Almond Sponge Cake Cream Roll, 45
Apricot Jam Filling, 55–56
Apricot Sauce for Duck or Chicken, 252–253
Artichoke Hearts, Baked, 193–194
Artificial sweeteners, 17
Atkins, Dr. Robert, 6–8
   Dr. Atkins' Diet Revolution, 6
   Dr. Atkins' New Carbohydrate Gram Counter, 6
   Dr. Atkins' New Diet Revolution, 8–9

Bacon, Spinach and Mushroom Salad, 212–213
Banana Cream Filling, 57
Banana Milk Shake, 95
Batter for Frying, 30
Beef:
   and Asparagus, Chinese, 234
   Boneless Roast, Herb-Crusted, 124–126
   and Broccoli, Chinese, 233–234
   buying, 16
   Cheese-Filled Hamburgers, 124
   with Chinese Vegetables, 236
   Japanese Grilled, 242–243
   Kebabs, 122
   Stroganoff, 123–124
   Sukiyaki, 244
   and Vegetable Salad, Chinese, 224–225
   See also Steak
Berry Misu, 84–85
Beverages, 6, 93–97
   See also Wines and liquors
Blackberry Jam Filling, 56
Blackberry Sauce for Duck or Chicken, 253–254
Blintzes, 53–54
Blitz diet, 4
Bluefish with Bacon, Broiled, 145–146
Borscht, Easy, 110
Borushek, Allan, *The Doctor's Pocket Calorie, Fat and Carbohydrate Counter,* 6

294   Index

Brandy Nut Kisses, 51–52
Brazil Nut Pie Crust, 46–47
Breads, rolls, and pancakes:
    Basic Noodle Dough, 39–40
    Batter for Frying, 30
    Blintzes, 53–54
    Cinnamon Bread, 33–34
    Cinnamon-Nut Coffee Cake Squares, 34–35
    Crêpes, 42–43, 54
    Easy-Mix Muffins, 31–32
    Easy-Mix Pancakes, 36–37
    French Toast, 38–39
    Herbed Rolls, 40–41
    Parmesan Puffs, 41
    Pecan Butter Coffee Cake, 35–36
    Puffy Pancakes, 37–38
Breakfasts, menus for, 11
Brown sugar, 17
Brunches, menus for, 11–12
Butter Sponge Cake Cream Roll, 43–44

Cabbage, Chinese Stuffed, 228–229
Cabbage, My Mother's Stuffed, 194–195
Cakes, 43–45, 55
    Fillings for, 57–62
    See also Coffee cakes
Calf's Liver, Sautéed, 140–141
Calorie-counting charts, 267, 268–292
Calorie-counting diets, 4
Calorie intake, controlling, as a diet, 4, 6
Carbohydrate gram-counting charts, 6, 267, 268–292
Carbohydrates, 5–6, 8

Cauliflower:
    Fried, 196–197
    with Cheese, 196
Caviar Omelet, 178–179
Celery:
    Braised Sliced, 197
    Gruyère, 198
Cheddar Scrambled Eggs, 175–176
Chef's Salad, 213
Cheese(s):
    and Herb Omelet, 180
    low-carbohydrate, 18
    Omelet, Double, 179
    Omelet, Italian, 185
    Sauce, 259
    Soufflé, 73–76, 188–189
    Spread, Nutted, 263
    Tomato, and Herb Omelet, 187–188
Cheesecakes:
    Marble, 65–66
    Refrigerator Banana, 67–68
    Refrigerator Italian, 66–67
    Refrigerator Lemon, 68–69
    Supreme, 64–65
Cherry Jam Filling, 56
Chicken, 159
    in Blue Cheese Sauce, 161
    Breasts, Baked Skinless and Boneless, 168
    Breasts, Curried, 165
    Breasts, Soy-Glazed, 164
    Broiled, aux Fines Herbes, 162
    Broiled, with Pesto, 168–169
    Broiled, with Shallot Butter, 159–60
    and Cauliflower, Chinese, 237
    with Cream and Herbs, 163
    Mustard Broiled, 160–161

Index

and Peppers, Chinese, 238
with Pesto and Ricotta, 167
Salad, Chinese, 223–224
Salad, Curried, 166
sauces for, 252–254
Sukiyaki, 244
Chicken-Liver Sauce, Steak with, 132–133
Chicken Liver Sauté, 166–167
Chinese dishes, 222–243
Chinese ingredients, low-carbohydrate, 18–19
Chives, 19–20
Chocolate:
 Almond Cream Filling, 61–62
 Almond Pie Filling or Pudding, 76
 Berry Soufflé, 73–74
 Egg Cream, 95–96
 Granite, 90
 Ice Cream, 86–87
 Mousse, 80–81
 Rum Cream Filling, 60–61
Cinnamon Bread, 33–34
Cinnamon-Nut Coffee Cake Squares, 34–35
Cinnamon-Pecan Puffins, 32–33
Cinnamon-Sugar Topping, 262
Clinical Nutrition, The American Journal of, 6
Coffee, 15
Coffee, Natalie's Iced, 96
Coffee cakes, 34–36
Coffee Granite, 89–90
Coffee Ice Cream, 87
Coffee Milk Shake, 94–95
Coleslaw, 214
Complete starvation diet, 3

Composition of Foods (USDA Handbook), 6
Consommé with Sherry, 108
Cookies, 51–52
Cooking, low-carbohydrate, tips for, 15–17
Cornish Hens, Glazed Rock, 170–171
Cornish Hens, Party, 172
Cornstarch, 20
Cranberry Sauce, Spiced, 252
Cream fillings for sponge cake rolls, 57–62
Cream of Tartar, 20
Crêpes:
 Flaming, 54
 Sweet, 42–43
Cucumber Salad, Sweet-and-Sour, 214–215
Cucumbers, Chinese Stuffed, 227–228
Curry (ied):
 Chicken Breasts, 165
 Chicken Salad, 166
 Eggs with Lobster, 177
 powder, 20
 Sauce for Seafood, 256–258

Dessert fillings, 55–62
Desserts:
 Berry Misu, 84–85
 Blintzes, 53–54
 Cakes, 43–45, 55
 Cheesecakes, 64–69
 Cookies, 51–52
 Crêpes, 42–43, 54
 Granites, 89–91
 Ice creams, 85–89
 Jelly Roll, 55
 Milk shakes, 93–96
 Mousses, 80–82

296 Index

Desserts (*cont'd*):
    Omelets, 70–73, 177–188
    Pies, 47–48
    Puddings, 76–82
    Soufflés, 73–75
    Stewed rhubarb, 69
    Strawberry shortcakes, 62–64
    Tiramisu, 82
Diet Pill Way, 4
Dieting, successful, tips on, 24–25
Diets, varieties of, 3–10
Dill, 20
Dinners, menus for, 12–14
Dr. Stillman's Quick-Weight-Loss Diet, 5
Drinking Man's Diet, The (Air Force Diet), 6
Duck, sauces for, 228–229, 252–254
Duck Sauce, Dietetic Chinese, 230

Easy-Mix Pancakes, 36–37
Edam Scrambled Eggs, 176
Egg Cream, Chocolate, 95–96
Egg Drop Soup, Chinese, 222
Eggplant Roll, My Mother's Stuffed, 198–199
Eggplant Slices, Broiled, 200
Eggs (and Egg Dishes), 20–21, 175–190
    Omelets, 70–73, 177–188
    Scrambled, 175–176
    Soufflés, 73–75, 188–190
Endive, Braised, 200–201
Escarole, Sautéed, 201
Extracts (flavoring), 21

Favorite Omelet, 180–181
Fines Herbes Omelet, 181
Fines Herbes Soufflé Omelet, 181
Fish:
    basic flavoring recipe for, 155
    Bluefish with Bacon, Broiled, 145–146
    buying, 15
    Mackerel, Spanish, Mustard-Flavored, 146
    Salmon Steaks, Grilled, with Anchovy Butter, 147
    Sesame-Crusted Tuna Fish, 154–155
    Shad en Papillote, 148
    Sole, Fillet of, with Parmesan Cheese, 154
    Sole Cordon Bleu, 149
    See also Seafood
Food Coloring, 21
Fredericks, *Dr. Carlton, Dr. Carlton Fredericks' Low-Carbohydrate Diet,* 6
French Toast, 38–39
Frio Frio, 92
Frozen Mochachino, 96–97
Fruits, low-carbohydrate, 15

Garlic and Parsley Sauce for Shrimp, 257–258
Gazpacho Soup, 119
Ginger juice, 21
Gingerroot, 21
Gingerbread Squares, 45–46
Gourmet Soufflé, 189
Granite:
    Chocolate, 90

Coffee, 89–90
Strawberry, 91
Greek Omelet, 182–183
Green Bean Salad, 215
Green Beans Amandine, 194
Green Peppers, My Mother's Stuffed, 203–205

Ham:
  and Cheese Omelet, 183
  -Mushroom Omelet, 184–185
  Omelet, 183
Hamburgers, Cheese-Filled, 124
Herbs, buying, 16
Herbs de Provence, 16
Herbed Rolls, 40–41
Hors d'oeuvre and appetizers, 100–117

Ice creams, 85–88
Ice Pops, 92–93
Ingredients for low-carbohydrate cooking, 17–24

Jam fillings for crêpes or rolls, 55–57
Jam Sandwich Cookies, 52
Jams, sugarless diet, 23
Japanese dishes, 242–247
Japanese ingredients, 18–19
Jelly Roll, 55

Lamb
  Chops or Steaks, Grilled with Mint Pesto, 138–139
  Herb-Crusted Leg of, 126–127
  Shish Kebab, 139–140
Lemon:
  Butter Cream Filling, 58
  Cake-Pudding, 78
  Chiffon Pie Filling or Pudding, 76–77
  Mousse, 81–82
  Pudding, 78–79
  -Sorrel Soup, Cold, 114–115
  Soufflé, Lovely, 74
  Soup, Frothy Greek, 113–114
  Sponge Cake Cream Roll, 43
Lime Chiffon Pie Filling or Pudding, 77–78
Liver, buying, 16
Liver Pâté, 101–102
Lobster, Curried Eggs with, 177
Lobster Tails, Broiled, 152–153
London Broil:
  with Boursin, 130
  Soy-Glazed, 131
Low-carbohydrate cooking ingredients, 17–24
Low-carbohydrate diets, advantages, 5–10
Lunches, menus for, 12

Mackerel, Mustard-Flavored Spanish, 146
Maple Walnut Cream Filling, 58
Maple Walnut Ice Cream, 87
Mayonnaise, 21
Mayo Clinic Diet (*Ten-Day Egg Diet*), 3
Mayonnaise Verte, 258
Meal frequency, greater, advantage of, 6

298 *Index*

Meat and Cheese Casserole, Italian, 127–128
Meat-Crusted Pizza, 128–129
Meats, 121
   Beef, 122–137, 224–225, 226–227, 228–229, 233–237, 242–243, 244
   Ham, 183–185
   Lamb, 128, 139–141
   Liver, 141–142
   Pork, 230–232
   Veal, 136–138
Melon with Prosciutto, 102–103
Melon Soup, Chilled, 115–116
Menus, sample low-carbohydrate, 11–14
Milk Shakes, 93–96
Mint Jelly, 254–255
Mint Pesto, 139
Mint Sauce, 255
Mousses, dessert, 80–82
Muffins, Easy-Mix, 31
   Variation, 32
Minster-Caraway Soufflé, 190
Mushroom(s):
   Chinese Stuffed, 225–226
   Creamed, with Cheese, 203
   Herbs, and Cheese Omelet, 186
   as low-carbohydrate ingredient, 22
   Salad, Bacon, Spinach and, 212–213
   Soufflé Omelet, 186–187
   Soup, Fresh-Hot or Cold, 111
   Stuffed, 105
Mustard Dressing, Beach House, 260–261
Mustard Sauce, Creamy, 259

Natalie's Iced Coffee, 96
Noodle Dough, Basic, 39–40
Nuts:
   Brandy Nut Kisses, 51–52
   Brazil Nut Pie Crust, 47
   Cinnamon-Nut Coffee Cake Squares, 34–35
   Nutted Cheese Spread, 263
   Pecan Butter Coffee Cake, 35–36

Oils for cooking, 22
Omelets, 177–188
   Dessert, 70–73
Onion Soup, French, 112
Orange:
   Brandied Cream Filling, 60
   Chocolate Cream Filling, 61
   Sponge Cake Cream Roll, 43

Pam non-stick product, 22
Pancakes, 36–38
   See also Blintzes and Crêpes
Parmesan Puffs, 41
Pasta, Mock, 202
Pecan Butter Coffee Cake, 35–36
Pepper(s):
   Chicken and, Chinese, 238
   Chinese Stuffed, 226–227
   and Mushrooms, Chinese Shrimp with, 241–242
   My Mother's Stuffed, 203–204
   Steak, Chinese, 235
Pesto Sauce, 262–263
Pie crusts, 47–48
Pies, *see* Puddings and pie fillings

Pizza, Meat-Crusted, 128–129
Poissonnade, 16
Pork:
  Chinese Barbecued
    Spareribs, 232–233
  Chinese Roast, 230–231
  and Cucumbers, Chinese,
    231–232
  See also Ham
Potato-like Salad, 216–217
  French, 217–218
Prosciutto, 22
  Melon with, 102–103
Puddings and pie fillings,
  76–82
Puffy Pancakes, 36–37
Pumpkin Soufflé, Frozen,
  74–75

Raspberry:
  Jam Filling, 56
  Soup, Cold Fresh, 116
  Sponge Pudding, 79–80
Rhubarb Sauce or Stewed
  Rhubarb, 69
Roquefort Dressing, 261
Roquefort Grapes, 104–105
Rumaki, 103

Salad Dressing, Chinese, 223
Salad dressing, buying, 16
Salade Niçoise, 210–211
Salads, 210–218
Salmon, Japanese Grilled
  (Salmon Teriyaki), 243
Salmon Salad Niçoise, Fresh,
  211–212
Salmon Steaks, Grilled, with
  Anchovy Butter, 147
Saturated fats, 7
Sauces, 251–263

Scampi, 151
Seafood:
  Chinese Barbecued Shrimp
    and Livers, 240
  Chinese Shrimp and
    Broccoli, 242–243
  Chinese Shrimp with
    Cucumbers, 240–241
  Chinese Shrimp Dip, 223
  Chinese Shrimp Egg Foo
    Yong, 238–239
  Chinese Shrimp with
    Peppers and
    Mushrooms, 241–242
  Curried Eggs with Lobster,
    177
  Curried Shrimp Salad, 152
  Curry Sauce for, 256
  Kebabs, 153–154
  Lobster Tails, Broiled,
    152–153
  Sauces for shrimp, 256–58
  Scampi, 150–151
  Shrimp Cocktails, 106; Hot,
    107
Shad en Papillote, 148
Shallots, 22
Sherry, 23
Shrimp:
  and Broccoli, Chinese,
    242
  Cocktails, 106; Hot, 107
  with Cucumbers, Chinese,
    240–241
  Dip, Chinese, 223
  Egg Foo Yong, Chinese,
    238–239
  Garlic and Parsley Sauce for,
    257–258
  and Livers, Chinese
    Barbecued, 240

300 Index

Shrimp (cont'd):
  with Peppers and Mushrooms, Chinese, 241–242
  Salad, Curried, 152
  Sauce, Dilled, 256–257
  Scampi, 150–151
Sole:
  Cordon Bleu, 149
  with Parmesan Cheese, Fillet of, 150
Soufflés, 182, 188–190
  Dessert, 73–75
Soups, 109–117, 222
South Beach Diet, 9
Soy flour, 23
  recipes for, 29–48
  Seasoned, 29–30
Spareribs, Chinese Barbecued, 204–205
Splenda®, 17
Spice Cake Cream Roll, 46
Spinach, Creamed, 205
Spinach, Sautéed, 206
Sponge Cake Cream Rolls:
  Banana, 57
  Chocolate Almond, 61
  Chocolate Rum, 60–61
  Lemon, 58
  Orange Brandied, 60
  Orange Chocolate, 61
  Maple Walnut, 58
  Strawberry, 59
  Vanilla, 59
Steak:
  buying, 16
  with Chicken-Liver Sauce, 133
  with Mushroom Sauce, 134
  Roquefort-topped, 132

Stock, chicken or beef, 23
Stracciatella Soup, 108–109
Strawberry:
  Cream Filling, 59
  Dessert Omelet, 72–73
  Granité, 90
  Ice Cream, 88–89
  Jam Filling, 56–57
  Shortcake, 62–63
  Shortcake, Individual, 63–64
  Soup, 116–117
Sukiyaki:
  Beef, 244
  Chicken, 245–246
  Vegetable, 247
Sweet Crêpes, 42–43
Sweet Pie Crust (Cookie Crust), 47–48
Sweet Puffy Omelet, 70–71
  Almond, 71
  Lemon, 71–72
Sweeteners, artificial, 17

Tea, 15
Ten-Day Egg Diet (*Mayo Clinic Diet*), 3
Tiramisu, 82
Tomatoes, Grilled, with Cheese, 206–207
Tuna Fish, Sesame-Crusted, 154–155
Turkey London Broil, Apricot-Glazed, 169–170
Turnips, French Fries, 207–208

Vanilla Cream Filling, 59
Vanilla Ice Cream, 85–86
Vanilla Milk Shake, 93–94
  Dietetic Variation, 94

Veal:
   Chops in Mustard Sauce, 137
   Scallops, Party, 136
   Scallops with Chives and Cheese, 135
Vegetable Sukiyaki, 247
Vegetables, 193–210, 227–229, 236
   Low-carbohydrate, 15
   See also Salads
Vinaigrette Dressing, 260
Vinegar, 23–24

Weight-Watchers Diet, 5
White Sauce, 251–252
Wine for cooking, 23, 24
Wines and liquors, carbohydrates in, 288–292

Zabaglione, 91–92
Zucchini:
   Bisque of, 113
   with Cheese, 210
   My Mother's Stuffed, 208–209